BREATHING
SPACES

NANCY N. CHEN

BREATHING SPACES

QIGONG,

PSYCHIATRY,

AND HEALING

IN CHINA

COLUMBIA UNIVERSITY PRESS
NEW YORK

COLUMBIA UNIVERSITY PRESS
Publishers Since 1893
New York   Chichester, West Sussex

© 2003 Columbia University Press

Library of Congress Cataloging-in-Publication Data
Breathing spaces : qigong, psychiatry, and healing in China /
    Nancy N. Chen
    p.   cm.
  Includes bibliographical references and index.
  ISBN 0–231–12804–5 (cloth : alk. paper) —
  ISBN 0–231–12805–3 (pbk. : alk. paper)
    1. Qi gong. 2. Qi gong — Political aspects. 3. Qi gong —
Social aspects. 4. Exercise therapy. 5. Psychiatry. I. Title:
Qigong, psychiatry, and healing in China. II. Chen, Nancy N.

RA781.8 .B73 2003
613.7'1 — dc21
                                            2002041121

Columbia University Press books are printed
on permanent and durable acid-free paper.

Printed in the United States of America
Designed by Lisa Hamm
c 10 9 8 7 6 5 4 3 2 1
p 10 9 8 7 6 5 4 3 2

FOR MY PARENTS

CONTENTS

PREFACE

BREATHE. *Imagine your breath as the way, taking the energy around you and combining it with your own energy. Relax. Exhale and empty yourself. Inhale and fill your being with the vitality of life. Visualize your qi energy as it circulates within your body and nourishes your inner organs. Open your senses to being in this universe.* These instructions came from a group of lively women in their fifties to seventies who met every day to practice this exercise together in Beijing. It was a familiar entry for anyone who has been introduced to the healing exercises known as qigong. Such instructions may sound exotic or mystical, but, like tai chi and yoga, qigong offered individuals the opportunity to engage in mind-body cultivation and healing. Through breathing exercises and visualization of qi (vital energy), qigong not only offered pleasurable somatic experiences but also generated new breathing spaces that transformed the contours of daily life.

In the post-Mao period, qigong flourished as a highly charismatic form of healing. I argue that the turn toward self-cultivation and alternative healing did not occur in a vacuum. Instead, as the Chinese state shifted from subsidized medicine to for-profit market medicine, qigong masters quickly assembled vast networks, across China and abroad, in response to concerns for health in the new economy. Three central arguments frame this ethnographic study. First, qigong was immensely popular mainly because it met people's needs to cope with chronic health concerns while promoting a sense of belonging. The transition to a market economy facilitated the widespread interest in qigong as an antidote through self-discipline. Second—less well known by most practitioners, especially outside China—qigong could potentially be harmful to certain individuals. The pathologies associated with the practice became medicalized into a new psychiatric category recognized by professionals. I document the unique ways in which qigong and psychiatry intersected for ordinary practitioners, certain patients, their families, work units, doctors, and bureaucrats. In tracing the transmission and travel of these forms of knowledge over a decade, my main focus is on the compelling search for healing found in both arenas. State officials initially promoted qigong because it was viewed as effective and uniquely Chinese. However, this shifted to regulation when certain masters were considered to be promoting pseudoscience. The boom period of widespread interest was curtailed by the active involvement of the state bureaucracy. Finally, the transnational travel of qigong masters and global followings disrupt any notions that qigong is solely a local Chinese practice unchanged by time.

By situating what took place in institutional settings within larger frameworks of social change in China, I hope to present a different view of the Chinese body politic, which tends to be portrayed as a hegemonic state operating though centralized planning and repressive control. Instead, this book examines moments when people came to embody and sometimes transform the state. The concept of body politics suggests that complex yet fluid interactions that take place among citizens, bureaucrats, and state institutions too often tend to be polemicized as a dichotomy between the people and the state. This ethnography offers a window for viewing the stories and experiences of ordinary people who participated in the qigong movement and lived in "interesting times."[1] While many texts now offer instructions on qigong forms of martial art or traditional healing, this book addresses the unique and relatively unknown intersection of qigong practice, psychiatry, and state policy.

Shortly after the meteoric rise of qigong practice, individuals complaining of a range of reactions, from mild discomfort and pain from qi or unusual sensations in their bodies to more dire sensations of hearing voices or being controlled by spirits and voices, began to trickle into traditional medical clinics and biomedical hospitals. My analysis of the relatively unknown culture-bound syndrome of qigong deviation is a key contribution. I examine how certain forms of experience related to qigong became medicalized in the psychiatric setting, in contrast to traditional medicine and cultivation practices. Narratives from patients, family members, and doctors are a crucial part of this discussion. Instead of solely focusing on psychiatry, I present material from noninstitutional sources to show how different notions of this disorder also circulated. My analysis addresses how not only qigong masters but also state media and popular texts were involved in the transmission of knowledge. Documenting the searches for healing that somehow became uncontrollable or mismanaged, leading eventually to hospitalization in psychiatric units, makes it possible to understand how notions of normality and mental illness were negotiated and defined. Tracing the gradual regulation of qigong healing and spiritual practices through the medicalization of qigong-related disorders also foregrounds current state regulation of alternative healing and spiritual cults. I analyze the evolving use of science as a way to contain the popularity of masters and maintain state order.

Spanning the decade of the 1990s, my research coincided with China's economic and social transformations during the late twentieth century. The fieldwork on psychiatry and qigong in China took place over one and a half years of research during 1990 and 1991. I undertook comparative research in Taiwan during the summer of 1992 and follow-up research in China in the fall of 1996. Later I conducted comparative work on qigong in the United States from 1995 to 1999. All names in this book have been changed to pseudonyms in order to maintain the confidentiality of psychiatric patients, qigong practitioners, family members, and doctors.

The reemergence of qi cultivation practices in the post-Mao context suggests the revival of alternative forms of healing and social order. *Breathing spaces* refers both to the literal experience of breath work and the production of spaces in all possible senses—phenomenological, social, and spatial—that emerged in qigong practice. By breathing deeply and slowly, either with others in unison or in solitary meditation, experiences of public spaces and urban sites could become infused with personal meaning and cosmological order rather than remaining solely official. Much has been written about the public sphere and emerging notions of citizenship over the past decade; however, such analyses leave out the ways in which feelings of belonging can be generated and literally incorporated into the body and one's sense of self. Contextualizing practices of self-making and cultivation can thus illuminate how a turn toward the self can be a political move rather than merely participation in narcissistic consumption. Personal and meaningful spaces for the self could be formed in the practice of qigong. These spaces were embodied by individuals and projected onto the human landscape despite a socialist urban context.

The diverse forms of qigong practice addressed so far indicate that qigong circulates in many different ways and contexts. Place is crucial to experience, and yet most discussions of qigong tend to focus on phenomenological aspects and address the flow of subjective experience. How are practices of self-cultivation transmitted in time and place? How do such practices transform the social and political context? In addition to discussing the practice of qigong in parks, this ethnography addresses the different social, institutional, and ideological locations of qigong practice, such as streets, auditoriums, work units, private clinics, state hospitals, and science discourses. The majority of ethnographic texts on China have either focused on ethnic minority groups or examined rural areas. This book is primarily based in urban China, in particular, its hospitals and parks. My purpose is to show how qigong is not just about healing: it also has political, entrepreneurial, and pragmatic dimensions.

Many texts of medical anthropology, specifically, the anthropology of psychiatry, question the boundaries of biomedicine. By showing the different social and political trajectories of qigong as alternative medicine in other places, I highlight how medicalization is a normative process that intimately links healers to the state, especially in postsocialist societies. Readers will come to appreciate that, though qigong tends to be portrayed as a traditional form of healing from China, such forms are much more pluralistic and politicized that what appears on the surface.

Writing as a medical anthropologist, I view the intersection of culture and medicine with a sense of great privilege and concern. Ethnomedicine, or the study of indigenous and traditional medicines, has long been a prominent category and the object of vigorous research in this field. Recent, more nuanced notions from literature characterized as critical medical anthropology have helped to reframe the divide between biomedicine and other forms of medicine to understanding biomedicine itself as a form of ethnomedicine. Moreover, a bifocal approach, where the ethnographer is attentive both to formations of institutional knowledge/power and their sites and to the lived experiences of individuals in such systems, offers rich possibilities for understanding the formation of subjects and alternatives in medicine, science, and technology.[2] Besides questioning categories and analyzing hierarchies of power, compelling ethnographic knowledge can offer insights into institutional and embodied practices.

Over the past decade, continued reforms to develop the Chinese market economy further have brought many structural and social changes, including the privatization of state-owned enterprises, commercialization of real estate, and heightened consumerism. The march toward World Treaty Organization (WTO) entry during the 1990s resulted in closures of factories, leading to unemployment and ongoing concerns about corruption and illegal migration. The emphasis on material life and consumption has been accompanied by profound social and spatial transformations as well. The fiftieth anniversary of the People's Republic of China (October 1, 1999) provided an opportunity for the Chinese leadership to celebrate elaborately China's transformation since revolutionary times. Any visible markers of social unrest or economic hardships, such as protesters and migrant workers, were systematically removed from all metropolitan areas. In Tiananmen Square, thousands of marchers and school-children joined the showcase of military prowess and weaponry. The carefully orchestrated display contrasted greatly with the volatile demonstrations that took place in the square a decade before, in 1989.

Over the past decade, qigong has expanded worldwide. I have been writing in Santa Cruz, California, another lively place of alternative healing and holis-tic medicine, where the search for healing reminds me how the desire for well-being is shared across cultures. Though the experiences of qigong practice can touch individuals regardless of cultural background, ultimately different con-texts create very different politics of healing. The controversial practice of falun-gong in China and its transnational presence evoke an eerie sense of déjà vu, raising parallels to the fervent support of qigong followers and the subsequent crackdown by the state. As I will address in this book, healing is a transforma-tive process similar to religious conversion. Many religious figures and charis-matic healers tell a common tale of suffering from illness and suddenly becom-ing transformed by healing powers. Medical and health practices are productive sites where we can see not just changing relations between the individual mind and body but also reflections of larger and highly charged relations between state and society. In my encounters with qigong practitioners, scientists, and bureaucrats, the same question—"Do you believe?"—was posed to me as a crit-ical point of entry. Such intense questioning reflected how one's location and frame of mind were crucial to understanding phenomenological experiences as well as ideological formations of the practice. Moreover, the passionate re-sponses to qigong practice and other forms of medicine by bureaucrats and by practitioners reveal how healing remains an inherently political act.

ACKNOWLEDGMENTS

THIS BOOK is the result of many collaborations and friendships over the years. I am deeply grateful to my mentors and colleagues in China. In particular, thanks to Professor Shen Yucun, who sponsored my initial study of families, social support, and psychiatric care. Special acknowledgement also goes to T. Zhang, Ellen Huang, Y. Zhong, Edward Shan, W. Hu, H. Zhang, and S. Nan for their invaluable help. Many patients, family members, and staff at the clinics and wards were generously supportive. Likewise, many healers and practitioners offered their assistance. While I cannot name them all and use pseudonyms in the text, I wish to express my continued gratitude and admiration to them.

My research and writing were supported by the Committee for Scholarly Communication with the People's Republic of China; the Institute of East Asian Studies, the Center for Chinese Studies, and the Department of Anthropology at UC Berkeley; the Jackson Kee Hu Memorial Scholarship and the Charlotte Newcombe Doctoral Dissertation Fellowship. A leave from the UCSC Department of Anthropology with support from the Division of Social Sciences and the Committee on Research at UC Santa Cruz enabled me to conduct follow-up research in 1995.

Writing can be a lonely process, but many people helped make the interminable task meaningful. Nancy Scheper Hughes, Frederic E. Wakeman, Laura Nader, Frank Johnson, Judith Justice, and Joyce Kallgren each offered important lessons that remain with me even now. My students in medical anthropology at UCSC and Tufts raised critical questions that help to frame this book. Feedback from colloquia organized by Hue-Tam Ho Tai and Stanley Tambiah at the John King Fairbanks Center at Harvard University and Jean Oi at the Institute of East Asian Studies of Stanford University were immensely useful. I am also grateful to Ann Anagnost, Jean Comaroff, Arthur Kleinman, Sue Naquin, Elizabeth J. Perry, Vivienne Shue, and Rob Weller for their incisive comments on papers presented at conferences.

The manuscript benefited immensely from the keen editorial eyes of colleagues, students, and friends. Steve Kurzman, Deborah Woo, and Raoul Birnbaum read a very early version. Jiemin Bao, Lesley Sharp, and Liu Yuan offered suggestions on the introduction. At different stages, I received invaluable comments from Fran Benson, Don Brenneis, Lawrence Cohen, Dana Frank, Milissa Gillen, Ann Kingsolver, Sing Lee, Dan Linger, Olga Najera Ramirez, Loki Pandey, Hugh Raffles, Carolyn Martin Shaw, Ken Shirriff, Alexandra Stern, Nigel Thompson, Rebecca Tolen, and Fred Wakeman. I am especially grateful to Bruce Grant and Nancy Ries, who swiftly read the manuscript in France and Moscow, respectively, and offered insightful suggestions. X. Zhang, J. Bao, and W. Hu offered advice on translations. Zoe Sodja helped with bibliographic sources. Just before the closure of the UCSC Document Publishing Center, Cheryl Van Der Veer found invaluable time to edit the manuscript as her last project there. Fred Deakin helped to incorporate her suggestions into the text. Sarah St. Onge copyedited the manuscript. I am deeply grateful to my editor, Wendy Lochner, and the two press reviewers whose belief in this book made it real.

The Ouyang, Zhang, and Lin families have warmly included me in their fold over the years, offering both moral and alimentary sustenance. The conviviality and support of friends also sustained this project. Thanks to Kathryn Barnard, Ken K. and Ann Beatty, Yuko and Akira Chiba, Gary Gray, Bill Handley, Terry Neudorf and Wei Wei, Pilar Owen, Annapurna Pandey, Darby L. Price, Indigo Som and Donna Ozawa, and Zhong Star. Dana Frank's offer of breathing lessons for swimming brought new insights to the meaning of breathing spaces. Special thanks to Sami for inspiring me to finish this project.

This book is dedicated to my parents, whose journeys in cultural translation enriched my own.

Santa Cruz, California

BREATHING
SPACES

CHAPTER ONE

INTRODUCTION

A DEEP BREATH of fresh air was always on my mind when I began field research on psychiatric practices and mental health care in Beijing during the winter of 1990. I lived in a high-rise apartment that faced similar gray buildings constructed in the 1950s. The smokestack of the building next door belched coal dust directly into my window, burning my lungs and making me wish for clear blue skies. Each morning I would look onto a solitary figure standing immobile on the opposite balcony. The whirring sound of pigeons circling nearby in the gray haze eerily accompanied this haunting image. I soon realized that this person's stance was part of a visualization practice in qigong, which required intense focus and simultaneous immersion in and withdrawal from the external world.

The quest for health, vitality, and longevity has been at the center of many spiritual and bodily practices in China for several millennia. Qigong is a form of healing and self-cultivation that reformulated traditional breathing and meditation techniques in the post-Mao reform period. A highly charismatic form of holistic healing, it eventually became regulated and reclaimed as state medicine. For a brief time, however, qigong flourished as a social and individual health pursuit avidly followed even by state officials. While I was conducting my research, the worlds of qigong and spiritual practice dramatically intersected with the worlds of science and bureaucracy in China. The bodily experience of qigong has been described by masters and lay practitioners as a force field or body of energy linked to natural forces. Visualization and imagination were central components in creating this body, which joined the individual senses and intellect to cosmological power. Commitment to daily practice brought agency in healing and new identities that embraced spiritual holism. The experience of practice in natural surroundings also renewed strong emotional links to an environment that could be reimagined to counter socialist urban anomie.

The tales of miraculous healing and other experiences that many practitioners described to me soon came to resonate with Mikhail Bulgakov's 1929 underground novel. *The Master and Margarita* takes place in a chaotic early Soviet system at the beginning of the twentieth century where good and evil engage in dialogue. Local citizens encounter mystical characters who test their morality and wreak havoc on those who succumb to greed. The insane asylum figures prominently in the novel as citizens are locked up when they claim to see the mystical figures. The novel's central characters include a petty bureaucrat, a mystical figure capable of shape shifting into animals and humans, and a young woman. As the lives of these characters become more closely interwoven, Bulgakov's critique of how socialist Russia had to contend with heterodox spirituality and even the shadow of Christianity emerges as a central motif.

The parallels with the social phenomenon of qigong deviation and political responses to this disorder were remarkable. Several prominent qigong masters claimed to have special mystical powers and attracted a wide following from all backgrounds, from factory workers to elite cadres. Names of ancient deities, Daoist practices of self-cultivation, and fantastic tales of superhuman abilities, which were suppressed as superstitious during the Cultural Revolution, resurfaced in public spaces and households. As the increasing influence of several masters became more apparent, state officials were quick to incarcerate one, declaring her to be a witch who profited from people's willingness to believe anything she said. Meanwhile, practitioners suffering from uncontrollable movements and visions related to qigong began to fill the psychiatric wards, complaining of losing control of the *qi* (chi) energy in their bodies. Many patients were brought in by families or work units after refusing food and claiming to be immortal or trying out their newly found healing abilities on others. After seeking help from traditional healers or medical doctors, families brought these patients to the hospital wards as a last resort.

This ethnography documents official and alternative practices of mental health in urban China. The ways in which individuals sought mental order through both orthodox biomedicine and alternative means of healing reveal responses to the tremendous economic and social transformations under market reform. In conversations with masters and lay practitioners of qigong, as well as with scientists and medical doctors, I was impressed with the sincerity with which people in these different realms sought order both personally and professionally. Though it would seem that the social worlds of qigong and a mental ward would be far apart, the intersections actually surfaced in surprising ways. My days began by watching my neighbor standing motionless on the balcony, continued with observing practitioners in the parks hugging trees, and ended with seeing patients in the mental hospital in the throes of uncontrollable qi energy, sometimes choking or bent over in pain. One hospital worker who was an avid follower of a female mystic whose career I will address in this book suddenly broke into uncontrollable sobs when our conversation turned to the fate of her newly imprisoned master. "Is she okay, have you heard from my teacher? She did nothing wrong. She is a true master." The worker's tears dried as suddenly as they came. Emotional and often passionate encounters such as these revealed how compelling the practice could become.

Despite the hazards of uncontrollable energy, qigong practice released the mind and body from the pressures of daily life in noninstitutional settings. For devoted practitioners, the exercises were moments of healing and transcendence over social or work obligations. Breathing spaces were carved out of the Chinese urban landscape of gray skyscrapers and busy streets through ecstatic experiences that took pleasure in the powers of healing and mental order.[1] Parks, courtyards, and even streets became spaces where it was all right to cry out or laugh uncontrollably. Mass qigong sessions, where a master would lecture and then heal individuals with internal energy, were strikingly reminiscent of spiritual revivalist movements in other cultural contexts and even political demonstrations of the Cultural Revolution. One master aptly concluded a group session of several hundred people by stating, "Qigong releases the soul of China." These occasions allowed members of the audience to experience spiritual transformations anonymously under the guidance of charismatic masters. Highly charged emotions were released with accompanying cries and tears of pain or pleasure as individuals were guided through sensory experiences. In the absence of strong religious institutions or emotional revolutionary campaigns after the Maoist era, gatherings of practitioners by the hundreds or thousands offered a social space for emotional and spiritual expression in a context of rapid urbanization and the shift to a market economy. Such gatherings were initially tolerated by the state, because participants emerged from them more productive, recharged, and revitalized.

Two ethnographic settings in China, the urban parks and the mental hospitals, situate the contradictory meanings of deviation and order that were eventually played out in public. My research was located inside Chinese mental hospitals in Beijing, Shanghai, and Laiyang (Shandong Province) as well as beyond the asylum in the parks of these cities. Set in a chronological window between the post-Tiananmen policies of 1990 and the revitalization of the Chinese economy in 1992, my examination of mental health care during this period focused on the relations between self-healing and institutional care. Later comparative research in Taiwan, the United States, and on the Internet allowed me to investigate the flows of practice and situated knowledges.

My role as an ethnographer emerged differently in the two research contexts. In the hospital, where the hierarchy of doctors, nurses, hospital staff, patients, and family members was visibly organized, I was introduced as a foreign researcher to all whom I encountered. In the parks, however, I began as an observer on early weekday mornings, from 6:30 A.M. to 8:00 A.M. This was the key time for many city residents to practice calisthenics, mass disco dance, strolling, tai chi, or qigong before going to work. The other major time for practitioners was Sunday mornings, the one free day before the institution of two-day weekends in 1995.

As city parks often drew people from all backgrounds, anyone who wished to participate in qigong could generally join in the morning sessions. Though speaking with strangers in other settings might be unusual, the common interest in qigong made it possible to strike up conversations quickly. In the course of such discussions, many practitioners would ask what form of qigong I practiced. I always responded that though I had studied other forms of martial arts since my teenage years, I did not yet practice or subscribe to any particular style of qigong. I was observing different methods for research. This exchange opened to me a world of practitioners who were eager to tell their stories of the search for healing and masters as well as to share inner experiences, which were ecstatic yet full of fearful apparitions.

The transformations that many people underwent in qigong practice paralleled my own journey as an anthropologist. Arriving in Beijing during the summer of 1985, I first lived and worked in China as an English teacher at the Beijing Institute of Iron and Steel Technology.[2] Like thousands of other "foreign experts" residing in China during the 1980s, I initially became immersed in Chinese social life and cultural politics through my students and colleagues and eventually through friends off campus. Their frequent stories about life during the Cultural Revolution (1966–1976) and views of Chinese modernization after Mao were interspersed with eager questions about American culture and life abroad. As the child of immigrant parents, raised in the United States, my life experiences were viewed as valuable if not instrumental.[3] Deeply moving stories about separation and struggles during the Cultural Revolution as well as about daily life in a new economic order led me to ask how families and different generations reworked their experiences of the past in the present. I had intended to study the role of family support in mental health care programs during graduate school.

The experiences and narratives of otherworldly journeys confronted me with the difficulty of writing an ethnography not only about life in a different country but about the problems of choosing the language with which to depict spiritual, social, and state discourses. Growing up in the southern United States, however, prepared me to examine spiritual aspects of healing in ways I did not expect. Qigong involves intense sensual engagement with the physical world as much as it entails disengagement from the social world where perceptions and the language of the senses are transformed. There is the difficulty of not only of translating Mandarin into English but also of making clear the culturally embedded meanings contained within psychiatric terms or descriptions of spiritual practices. How does one describe the sensations of orienting oneself to the cosmological world while also having a physical body with familial and institutional ties? How does one describe the mind-body experience of having inner and outer worlds collapse, allowing the chaos within oneself and in the social context to be embraced? These were extraordinary experiences of ordinary people: street sweepers, factory workers, bike lot attendants, students, professionals, even bureaucrats, who were playing with the boundaries of mind-body and experiencing other realms of reality where qi energy became the main source of spiritual and physical nourishment.

The role of an anthropologist as outsider to another culture has been effectively problematized by the literature on "halfies" or "native" anthropologists (Narayan 1997; Navaro-Yashin 2002; Altorki and El-Solh 1988). In writing about technologies of the self in craft making, Dorinne Kondo (1991) also addressed her own identity as both insider and outsider in Japanese society. Her vivid account of viewing the reflection of a Japanese woman in a department store window and suddenly realizing that it was actually herself brought to the surface the issue of what it meant to be a *sansei*, or third-generation Japanese-American ethnographer in Japan. My own location as a second (or 1.5)-generation Chinese American was often folded into the category of the returning overseas Chinese for whom going home had an extensive social meaning. Returning in my case resonated with an additional layer of meaning as I had already lived and worked in China as an English teacher for several years before returning as an anthropologist. I was accepted in my encounters at the hospital, in the parks, and on the street not solely because of perceptions of shared Chineseness but also because of my identity as a research scholar, which had a special significance in both the medical and qigong communities. The confluence of being a Chinese American ethnographer in both contexts led to moments of serendipity in which my difference and sameness mattered greatly.

In what follows, I address four contexts that frame this study of qigong. I begin with the spiritual and medical traditions in China that form the roots of qigong. There are multiple notions of qigong, not only because there are different forms of qi but also because of the contemporary proliferation of the practice. There was an incipient phase of interest in qigong during the early socialist era of the 1950s. This was followed with a quick demise when the Maoist state used antisuperstition campaigns to mobilize against *yiquandao* (way of basic unity) sects. I then turn to examining qigong from the perspective of medical anthropology and psychiatry. Finally, I address how qigong branched out in the transnational context as an extension of alternative medicine. Alternative medicine tends to be addressed in a celebratory fashion without much regard for historical context. The return of qigong in this context seemed familiar but was quite different during the 1990s.

LOCATING QIGONG

Qigong is a health practice that involves breathing, mental imagery, and sometimes movement. The term "qigong" has been translated in several ways according to notions of qi as air, breath, energy, or primordial life source. According to Liu and Wu's [1990a–f] multivolume study of qi across eight dynasties, qi—also known as *chi* or *ki*—is neither matter nor spirit but the primordial source of all life. *Gong* refers to the skillful movement, work, or exercise of the qi. It is the root used in words referring to martial arts such as *gongfu* (*kungfu*) and further invokes a sense of achievement, service, or ability, used in terms such as *gongde* (meritorious deeds), *gongfu* (ability or skill), *gongke* (homework), and *gongming* (scholarly honor or rank). The physical manifestation of qi has often been described as warm and located at the center of the body. As a bodily exercise, the practice relies on breathing exercises to attain vast transformations in one's state of mind and health. As a meditative practice, visualization of energy facilitates the integration of mind, body, and spirit with oneself and one's environment. Movement, too, is sometimes involved.

In China, qigong is linked to a wide spectrum of practices ranging from self-cultivation, meditation, medical healing, and breathing to martial arts, each with a specific history and genealogy. As there are literally hundreds, even thousands of forms, tracing the lineages of qigong can be an elusive and even Sisyphean task. To help frame the ensuing discussion, I draw on the image of a giant living tree with deep extensive roots and multiple branches. The metaphor comes from my field research in parks, where trees were integral to the daily practice of many practitioners whom I observed and interviewed. Arboreal metaphors were frequently invoked not only at the personal level to describe the experience of related knowledge but also at the transnational level to describe the connectedness between local and overseas Chinese.[4]

Though many masters and texts claim that qigong is over five thousand years old, several scholars and masters consider the term to be of recent vintage, less than a century old by some accounts (Xu 1999). A common origin story told to me by scholars was that qigong was a project sponsored by the Communist Party. The term "qigong" itself was a neologism, nonexistent before the 1950s. The notion of qi and existence of qi cultivation exercises, however, have been documented in numerous medical texts and spiritual practice traditions for several millennia (Englehardt 1989). Traditional Chinese medical, spiritual, and philosophical traditions form the extensive roots of knowledge about qigong, while contemporary extensions of qigong include numerous martial arts forms, spiritual practice spinoffs, and newly regulated scientific qigong. Qigong is different from *taijiquan* and *gongfu* in that it is not solely a martial art form. It is also a healing art that can be practiced by masters on patients who are nonpractitioners. Despite the multiple forms and styles of qigong, nearly all practitioners and masters acknowledge its revitalizing effects for the mind, body, and spirit as well as the potential for enhancing potency and longevity. One way to distinguish among the different forms or styles is through movement. Certain forms tend to be introspective and meditative (*nei gong*) for the practitioner, while other forms tend to focus on external energy and motion (*wai gong*). Kenneth Cohen, an American qigong master, describes these as "dynamic or active qigong (*dong gong*) and tranquil or passive qigong (*jing gong*)" (1997, 4). Another way of categorizing the various forms of qigong differentiates them according to the arenas of spiritual practice, martial arts, and medical healing traditions that incorporate qi cultivation or breathing exercises.

The traditional practices of cultivation perhaps most closely linked to qigong exercise are Daoist forms of breathing and internal transformation. Cultivation, the training of one's mind and body to refine the self, lies at the heart of most indigenous Chinese body practices. At the heart of Daoism, however, there is also the belief in qi as primordial and preexisting before all other forms of life. It is important to note that Daoist practices are also quite heterogeneous because of the multiple schools that emerged over the centuries (*Laughing at the Tao* 1995). Different texts, rituals, and movements have been described as Daoist but might actually be related only marginally. Many breathing exercises were secularized and practiced not only by Daoists but by Buddhists and medical practitioners as well. Contemporary qigong practitioners and scholars also invoke Daoist beliefs about cultivation and visualization. At the heart of Daoism, however, was the belief in qi as primordial and preexisting before all other forms of life.

Cultivating qi on an individual basis involves transcending one's everyday thoughts and perceptions to facilitate opening up to a larger cosmological order via breathing. Daoist cultivation practices have for centuries focused on breathing as a tool for internal alchemical changes in the quest for immortality (*Laughing at the Tao* 1995; Schipper 1993). A common precept urged practitioners to focus on breathing techniques: "Do not listen with your ears or heart-mind (*xin*) but with the breath" (Robinet 1997, 35). In two central Daoist texts, the *Taipingjing* and the *Huangtingjing*, the process of meditation involves deep visualization of one's own viscera and breath in order to renew and transform the body. While Daoist body transformations focus primarily on internal alchemy for the ultimate goal of immortality, qigong promotes both internal cultivation and external bodily strength. At the very core of qigong and other cultivation practices, breath and the movement of vital energy through one's body have been the central principle of connecting body, self, and environment.

In many indigenous cultures and traditional medical systems, the process of breathing and the external environment of air and wind were viewed as a continuum. The movement of air was viewed as a sacred power. The significance of breath for both physical animation and well-being has been noted by scholars and practitioners alike. In his tracing of the elements responsible for life itself—pulse, blood, and respiration—in ancient Greek and Chinese medicinal systems, Shigehisa Kuriyama asserted that the Chinese emphasis on breath (qi) was a major point of divergence from Western practice (1999, 6). Though Greek medicine shared similar concepts of humoral theory, even linking wind to certain pathological states, traditional Chinese medicine eventually developed a much more elaborate framework that linked forms of breathing to states of health. Although respiration can be conceived of as a mechanical process, breathing practices are considered to be the foundation for spiritual and physical healing.

It is easy to take this very primordial and simple function for granted. The importance of breathing is more often marked by its absence or anomalies. For instance, among individuals who experience reduced capacities for breathing, because of blocked sinuses during a cold or chronic asthma, it is only when breathing is restored that the connection between breath and wellness is fully appreciated.[5] In his analysis of the classification of pathology, George Canguilhem provocatively stated, "Respiratory rhythm is a function of our awareness of being in the world" (1989, 168). To elucidate the linkages among self, emotion, and society, Margot Lyon addressed how respiration is "implicated in the generation and experience of emotion in the social context" (1994, 84). Though breathing is determined by both autonomic and voluntary control, subjective variations in respiratory rhythm and form are characteristic of many shamanic or ritual trance states as well as clinical pathological states such as panic attacks or hyperventilation. Lyon further points out that patterns of breathing are very adaptable and can form a bodily environment structured by individual emotion.

It was in the course of observing daily qigong practices that I learned about the different ways people breathe and the many forms, patterns, and rhythms of breath. Rather than instructing people to breathe with their noses, masters and practitioners explained to them how to breathe through their bodies, especially through the internal organs, such as the kidney or spleen, sites of important concepts in traditional Chinese medicine. In contrast to states of fear and heightened arousal, where breathing is shallow or even withheld, the healing breaths in qigong emphasized deep breathing from the center of one's body. Deep respiratory rhythms combined with meditative visualization in tune with the landscape could easily transform a practitioner's sensory perceptions. Many practitioners claimed they could be healed of chronic ailments and even heal others with their newly enhanced powers simply by altering their breathing. It was from narratives of practitioners that I learned about the power of breath and the consequences of improper breathing. Yet, in the process of reordering space and time according to one's own respiratory rhythms, it was also possible to induce deviant patterns that generated further disorder.

Certain martial art forms of qigong utilized breathing to strengthen and push the body to extreme limits.[6] Martial arts and acrobatic movements are found in many classic Chinese operas and contemporary novels (*wuxia xiaoshuo*). Often performing in public, on streets or at festivals, masters would engage in incredible demonstrations of invulnerability to blows, piercings, or even fire. Two frames from *San Mao Liulangji* (San Mao vagrant chronicles), a widely popular cartoon series from the 1920s, shows the hapless fate of San Mao, Zhang Leping's street urchin hero, when assisting a martial arts performer. In "Tongshi ertong" (Everyone's child; see fig. 1a), a large crowd of kids and their families looks on while San Mao is twisted into a contorted pose. In "Baimai liqi" (Waste of strength; see fig. 1b), another crowd watches while San Mao laboriously performs more feats, only to disperse quickly when a collection plate is circulated.

The emphasis on transcending limits of pain and carrying out superhuman tasks in such forms of qigong appealed greatly to organizations that trained followers in military fashion. In 1918 the Republican government promoted "new martial arts" as part of the *guocui* (national essence) movement (Brownell 1995, 53). Over the next decade, the revival of martial arts was linked to growing nationalism. In writing about the "new martial arts" or

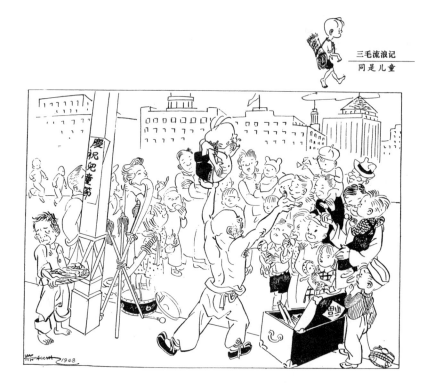

IA. Depictions of external qi and martial arts street performances in early-twentieth-century Shanghai. *"Tong shi ertong" (Everyone is a child)*. SOURCE: Zhang Leping, *San Mao Liulanji*.

"Chinese-style gymnastics," writer and social critic Lu Xun pointed out that such exercises have two main functions: physical education and military training (cited in P. Cohen 1997, 230). He cautioned, however, against the "feudal superstition" that such arts promoted (cited in Brownell 1995, 53). Even today, certain martial art forms of external qigong continue to be taught as basic military training. Such forms are believed to be ideal ways to prepare for conditions such as thirst, hunger, and pain that may be experienced in combat or in extreme environments.

Most Chinese sectarian uprisings and rebel movements in the past have included some form of physical regimen or martial arts movements involving qi.[7] Qigong or breathing exercises seemed to be a fundamental building block not

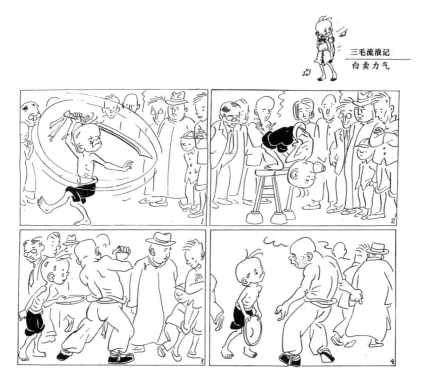

1B. Depictions of external qi and martial arts street performances
in early-twentieth-century Shanghai. *"Baimai liqi" (Waste of strength).*
SOURCE: Zhang Leping, *San Mao Liulanji.*

only for spiritual cults but also for peasant resistance. The draw to such groups
and their rapid spread across different regions during moments of political unrest could be attributed to several factors: a keen sense of invulnerability and
power from personally experiencing qi, the forging of social identity and connection with larger networks beyond family and village, and, ultimately, transformations of peripheral status to inclusion within a social movement.

Scholars of Chinese secret societies and millenarian movements have frequently noted the use of qi exercises by sect leaders and their followers as part
of induction rituals and martial arts training. Qigong and qi cultivation were
part of regimens intended to strengthen the bodies and minds of followers
within the larger order of sectarian organizations. Official documentation in-

dicates that Boxers and White Lotus members incorporated daily regimens of martial art movements as well as breathing exercises to enhance their qi.[8] Susan Naquin's study of the heterodox White Lotus sects in northern China focused on the 1774 Shantung uprising led by Wang Lun during the mid–Qing dynasty. In training exercises, the leader learned special mantras and techniques of fasting, meditation, and boxing that bear a striking resemblance to contemporary forms and movements. The "mastery of techniques of fighting, meditation, drinking 'purified water,' and going without food, and membership in the sect were the keys to survival" (1976, 59). Similarly members of the Boxer Uprising (1898–1900), at the dawn of the twentieth century, incorporated "hard (*ying*) form of deep breathing exercise (qigong) accompanied by the recitation of magical formulas and the swallowing of charms" (P. Cohen 1997, 101). Such forms were believed to lead to experiences of spirit possession that ultimately could make followers invulnerable to all opponents and their weapons. The magistrate Ji Gui-jen in 1899 recorded the following statement about a Shaolin monk who helped to train Boxers "My whole body has qigong; I can resist spears and guns" (Esherick 1987, 225). These brief glimpses of cultivation practices documented in official records suggest that breathing exercises were integral to the formation and military training of sectarian groups.

Though Shaolin forms of martial arts include dramatic feats of physical strength and prowess, most Buddhist practices of cultivation mainly emphasize meditation and internal forms of qi transformation crucial to enhancing one's spiritual development. In contrast to Daoist practices, which focus intensively on bodily cultivation for longevity and potency, regimens of the body in Buddhist practice address transcendence of bodily constraints. Nonetheless, sinicized Buddhism was influenced by and even incorporates Daoist practices. For instance, certain breathing exercises and physical movements such as *yijingjing* are used by monks to prepare for long periods of stillness and deep meditation. Buddhist qigong also tends to emphasize healing as an integral part of the spiritual process (Birnbaum 1989). The presence of qi used to nurture the body corresponds to frequent depictions of Buddhas with expansive bellies. Rather than being the result of extreme consumption of food, such girth was due to the daily regimen of qi exercises that promoted spiritual growth and power emanating from the center of the body.

In Chinese traditional medical knowledge, breath is viewed as a manifestation of one's qi or vital energy. While the corporeal body in contemporary Chinese medicine has been anatomized and embedded in the physical world, the energetic body signified by qi energy suggests links to cosmological entities beyond this world (Farquhar 1994). Early anatomical drawings from traditional medical texts describe the center of the body as the sea of qi (*qi hai*). Such mappings of the body remain deeply embedded in the mentalities of practitioners, especially those engaged in healing. In medical texts such as the *Huangdi Neijing Suwen* (*Yellow Emperor's Canon of Internal Medicine*), qi was a primary organizing principle and element of the human body. Most traditional Chinese medicine (TCM) techniques such as acupuncture, moxibustion, massage, and herbal remedies are utilized to animate the qi, which may be stagnant or pathological.

In the middle of the twentieth century, the integration and codification of TCM into a state system of socialist medicine meant a reorganization of theories of the body and medical healing. Qigong managed to be incorporated and preserved as a form of traditional medical practice (Hsu 1999). This ideological and literal location in TCM enabled medical qigong to survive, even as old feudal and superstitious practices were purged later in the 1960s and 1970s during the Cultural Revolution.[9] In the 1990s manuals that discussed different forms of breathing and qi exercises openly circulated as personal handwritten copies and new publications in state bookstores.

BODIES, SPACES, AND CULTIVATION

Critical medical anthropology has always engaged with body politics through examination of how medical institutions shape knowledge and regulation of the body. The growing literature from this perspective addresses how bodies are embedded within complex matrices of social and political institutions (Turner 1996). Foucault's early work on discipline and his later project on care of the self both evoke cultivation as a component of the processes of discipline and care. Thinking with the body illustrates how hegemonic institutions come to reside in the very core of one's physical being and environment. A significant link between bodies and spaces was elaborated early by Foucault in his study of the clinic and the role of the medical gaze in establishing pathology: "Clinical experience sees a new space opening up before it: the tangible space of the body, which at the same time is that opaque mass in which secrets, invisible lesions, and the very mystery of origins lie hidden" (1994, 123). The human body in his view was a set of spatialized knowledge in which disease could be mapped out with patterns, "forms and seasons that [a]re alien to the space of societies" (16). Seeing and entering the body in this way generated new structures of knowledge independent of the social systems that previously circumscribed the natural body. His insistence on the "contrast between a medicine of pathological spaces and a medicine of the social space," however, reflected a desire for healing that did not rely on the configuration of disease within bodies (38).

Prompted by such hopes for more social forms of medicine, I consider the ways in which bodies and spaces can be mutually constitutive in clinical contexts and practices of self-cultivation, which both offer very different social and political possibilities for embodiment and agency. One set of spaces was created by state institutions as part of an ongoing commitment to mental health and public hygiene. Clinical practices of psychiatry offered families and work units much-needed arenas within which to address mental illness and social disruption while maintaining a sense of order. The other set of spaces was tied to extraordinary material and social changes associated with market reforms that gave rise to new options in social life often characterized as civil society that could serve as popular alternatives to state formations. The breathing spaces cultivated by individual practitioners in new social formations opened possibilities for healing experiences and networking beyond state formations. Through alternative healing and imagining the breath, the practice of qigong also transformed the individual's spatial and temporal relations. The body was not only embedded within the physical world but also a natural symbol of cosmological power.

Over the past two decades, the body has been the locus of cultural and political struggles as well as a springboard for social theory. In anthropology, the body has been a rich source of cultural metaphors and the focus of critical analysis. Drawing on John O'Neill's initial exploration in an essay of great relevance to medical anthropology, Nancy Scheper-Hughes and Margaret Lock (1987) identified three bodies with overlapping arenas of experience related to sickness or disease.[10] In their reframing, which challenged the legacy of dualism, the individual body was the lived body of the self and the corporeal entity that experiences health and illness. The social body was not only a collective entity but also the arena where representations and symbolic meanings of disease can be inferred. The body politic was the continuum of the individual and social bodies where "regulation, surveillance, and control" are exerted (27). This third metaphorical sketch of the body was an early attempt to align with Foucault's project of biopower, where institutional power becomes diffused and internalized in corporeal bodies. Instead of representing space as an empty void, Foucault (1973) suggested in his concept of biopower that the spatial arrangements of particular institutions such as prisons, schools, and factories were instrumental to the reproduction of institutional power. Bodies were the literal product of such spatial arrangements and necessary for the reproduction of power. Such a notion of the body politic went beyond more direct notions in which a ruler is literally the head of state while ministers or generals are various appendages of the national body.[11] Instead, this third sense of the body politic offered ways to think about institutions and their subjects simultaneously. The social spaces created by state projects in particular reflect geographies of power that individuals must negotiate. Lefebvre's (1991) analysis of the production of space also cautions against thinking solely in terms of spatiality. His project of uncovering the social relations inherent in spaces has helped to broaden my understanding of embodiment as a particular placement of power relations. Extending Lefebvre's analysis to the production of gender, feminist urban theorists such as Massey and Rose have noted that spaces are not simply passive conduits of state power but also arenas of active social relations and movement in time (Massey 1994, 94; Rose 1993).[12] The concept of body politics is a useful analogy to understand the rather divergent directions in which social support of qigong challenged the state and yet qigong discourse was incorporated and used to promote official ideology.

Over the past decade several scholars have focused on affliction and suffering. In doing so, the analytical gaze has been broadened from the centers of knowledge and production to the production of difference and deviance in illness, sickness, and disease (Kleinman, Das, and Lock 1997; Scheper-Hughes 1992). The power of postcolonial and global economies to produce working bodies within iatrogenic conditions of "illth"(Frankenburg 1992) and violence as opposed to health have been extensively documented in ethnographies by Comaroff (1985), Taussig (1987), Scheper-Hughes (1992), and Farmer (1992). Explorations of body politics reveal a continuous relationship between individuals and medical and state institutions. Each of these analyses has been foundational in mapping relations between bodies and regulatory states. In her essay "The End of the Body?" Emily Martin (1992) queried the heightened focus on the body and its centrality as a social form in the late twentieth century. In tracing the transition from a notion of the body as fixed and predictable as part of Fordist mass production to the more flexible bodies needed for mass accumulation in global markets, Martin succinctly addressed the deeply felt cultural anxieties about changing boundaries of the corporeal body as a necessary end. Toward the end of the twentieth century and even in the beginning of the twenty-first century, the fascination with bodies has deeply resonated in popular culture. Feminist and other scholars have for decades revealed the power of political discourses such as gender, sexuality, and race to shape bodies (Balsamo 1996; Grosz 1994). Body images promoted in body building, fashion, advertising, and even children's toys reflect an obsession with bodies and their malleability.

A central issue that I am concerned with is whether political order or institutions can be reconfigured with practices that involve changes in body regimen and order. Though the body is a site of discipline and containment, it can also be a site of resistance. The literature on trance, possession, and ecstatic states has persuasively suggested how bodies can become unbound from state and social regulation by experiences of illness and in extreme cases even possession (Sharp 1993). Subversion of discipline through indigenous belief and practice has been explored through Comaroff's (1985) work on Christianity and Ong's (1987) work on Malay spirit possession in Japanese-owned factories. Such resistance, either indirectly or openly expressed, is often read by anthropologists as an embodied response to the violence of everyday life in situations where lives are endangered, threatened, and compromised by shocking and continuous invasions of the state into personal life (Taussig 1992). Understanding resistance and transgression offers a double view, not only of instances where the mind-body becomes unbound but also a wider perspective of moments when the state reconstitutes itself through violent modes of discipline. Agency in healing can thus be at once empowering and socially disruptive. This has led me to explore practices that nurture self-cultivation, which may not only promote breathing room apart from institutional time and space but even have the potential to undo official state agendas.

Knowledge of the body is constructed and regulated by medical institutions, whether in Asian medical systems or in biomedical settings (Lock 1993; Martin 1994; Turner 1996). Two organizing principles with distinctly different views of the body can be found in biomedical and traditional forms of medicine. In biomedicine, the anatomical body is the site of practice for medical institutions, such that healing focuses primarily on corporeal treatments. In traditional Chinese medicine, as well as in other medical traditions, the mind-body distinction is less meaningful. Instead, the dualistic entities of *nei* (internal) and *wai* (external) have more dynamic implications for the mind and energetic body. While the three-bodies approach illustrates the layers of power that define individual experiences of health and illness, an anthropological understanding of bodies must consider the appeal of spiritual holism, which links the inner and outer dimensions of the mind and body.

The notions of an inner body and external body are found not only in canons of traditional Chinese medicine but also in traditions of folk healing alternative to state medicine. Chinese spiritual traditions have tended to emphasize the inner world of spiritual experience, where practice develops one's capability to move from being in the world to other realms. Daoist and other forms of healing focus primarily on the spiritual realm, such mind and spirit are integrated in the body. Daoist alchemy focused on the active restructuring of inner elements with mental and bodily practices. Inner mystical experience, particularly in Daoist healing, emphasized dimensions beyond the reach of state discourse (Kohn 1992; Schipper 1993). It is precisely this notion of the inner body and mind transformed through spiritual practice that offers possibilities of transcendence beyond state bodies and institutions of power. Cultivating one's qi involves a leap of faith from the physical and social world to inner worlds of experience as part of metaphysical transformation. Practitioners often talked about achieving freedom through one's mind and spirit rather than remaining in the everyday world with one's body.[13]

Though traditional medicine tends to be valorized as an alternative to biomedicine in North America, it is crucial to remember that in the People's Republic of China (PRC), traditional Chinese medicine is quite integral to state medicine. Chinese medical institutions also view the individual mind-body as an integral part of the state corpus (Unschuld 1985; Sivin 1995a). Bodily organs are likened to state bureaucrats both in terms of both function and their relationships with each other. During the Republican era (1911–1949), the hygiene movement focused on public health. In the early years of socialist medicine, health was the responsibility of the government, such that healing was both a political platform and subject to state regulation. The socialist vision of healthy bodies follows a longstanding Chinese political movement in the twentieth century to counter stereotypes of the "sick man of Asia." Under Mao, all schools, factories, and prisons had daily morning exercises. The leader's body was also the site of intense scrutiny. When Mao swam across the Yangzi River, it was celebrated as a feat of strength and resolution. State medicine idealizes the cultivation of healthy, functioning bodies for efficient production. Disciplined and healthy bodies are viewed as the primary building blocks for nation building and the image of the Chinese socialist state. China's planned-birth policy in particular has been a key example of the production and surveillance of bodies in post-Mao China (Anagnost 1997). Susan Brownell's (1995) ethnography of Chinese athletes explores the notion of body culture, which incorporates concepts of body techniques by Mauss, habitus and practice by Bourdieu, and micro techniques of discipline from Foucault. Broadly defined as all forms of "embodied practice" including "daily practices of health, hygiene, fitness, beauty, dress, and decoration, as well as gestures, postures, manners, ways of speaking and eating, and so on," the concept of body culture is an intervention in the literature that focuses solely on phenomenological experience as the way to understand how bodies both experience and inhabit the world (10).

The density of urban life generated many feature stories in the Chinese media during the post-Mao years. A report on crowded buses on the main newswire stated that the average bus in Shanghai in the 1980s carried up to ten persons per square meter on average. On long daily commutes across town, I experienced the sheer physicality of squeezing into an old metal bus with several hundred other passengers. On popular routes oncoming passengers often collided with those trying desperately to get off at their stop. It was not unusual to have one's whole body pressed into others, all the passengers unified as an amoebic mass, simultaneously jostled as the bus lurched forward or jerked to a halt. In such spatial arrangements, most urban residents were mindful of both physical meanings as well as social and political notions of spaces. There was a very strongly felt need for physical space, for which practices of self-cultivation in parks were a partial response, providing urban relief.

Though traditional Daoist cultivation practices involved rituals of breathing, meditation, and fasting, contemporary notions of cultivation can include a wider range of practices that incorporate more recent technologies of leisure and self-improvement. On daily visits to parks, one would see mostly elderly retirees walking briskly on sidewalks or leaning against fences to stretch their legs. Nearby, in pavilions or open concrete spaces, groups of middle-aged couples would waltz or tango to strains of concert music from a single tape player. Even louder disco music broadcast from park speakers accompanied large groups of fifty to seventy people, mostly women, as they danced to Bananarama and Madonna. In more quiet and isolated pockets of city parks, one could easily spot schools of *taiji* (tai chi) and qigong practitioners. Taiji was usually presented as a form of group exercise, while qigong more openly invoked spiritual cultivation and miraculous healing, its adherents more eclectic in their practice. Smaller groups of a dozen people would participate in group meditation and healing sessions, while individuals could also be found in isolated spots of meditating quietly or vigorously motioning to bring the qi of special trees into their being. In such daily practices, individuals seeking healing or meditation not only occupied public spaces, but such spaces also promoted the cultivation of certain bodies and social relations.

A crucial anchor of this book is concerned with the ways in which practices of self-cultivation in certain times and places enabled the transformations of existing spaces and even transcendence of spatial and institutional boundaries. In his final volume of *The History of Sexuality*, Foucault (1986) turned to the study of ancient Greek moral systems and the economy of pleasure that subsequently emerged. The turn to care of the self and new modes of personal conduct, he argued, was not a result of a strong civic or public authority "but rather a weakening of the political and social framework within which the lives of individuals used to unfold" (41). Cultivating the self and the body was a reflection not merely of individual pursuits but "came to constitute a social practice, giving rise to relationships between individuals, to exchanges and communication, and at times even to institutions" (45). In other words, practices of self-cultivation were powerful techniques with generative effects capable of transforming not just personal regimens but also political entities.

The body can thus be viewed as a nexus that enables alternative forms of political engagement. Following the work of critical medical anthropologists and feminist scholars who have problematized boundaries between the private and public spheres, I consider breathing spaces in qigong to be productive sites where new possibilities for collective experience were forged. Such spaces were not only the literal locations where practices took place but also ephemeral moments in which alternate modalities of being and experience could be generated. For instance, mass qigong sessions were temporary gatherings, yet participants reported experiencing long-lasting effects. The transformation of spatial and temporal boundaries of the work unit, state media, and streets in China was far-reaching.

The political and economic context in which qigong emerged serves not only as a backdrop but as a critical point of enquiry about body politics. Emily Martin's (1994) analysis of the immune system provides useful clues for understanding what is at stake in contestations over the popular practice of qigong. Martin linked the biomedical constructions of the inner body with the external formations and constraints of late capitalism. Particularly in corporate America, where workers are increasingly expected to be flexible—that is, prepared to accommodate the whims and movement of global capital—she found an analogous production of new subjectivities in biomedicine. China's embrace of global capitalism, which meant the opening of international market forces abroad and the adoption of market economies at home, gained momentum during the 1980s and proceeded with renewed force in the mid-1990s. As the Chinese government mobilized in preparation for the WTO during the late 1990s, there have been massive layoffs of factory workers and deepened inequalities between rural and urban regions. Socialist medicine was also downsized as the health benefits that mostly urban residents depended on were cut during reconstructions of state funding. At the time of its reemergence, qigong provided an alternate space and opportunities to imagine and experience daily life. Moreover, the embrace of alternative health care in the post-Mao period reflected that somehow not all forms of illness or disease could be addressed by state institutions of health care. Qigong was promoted by masters and bureaucrats alike as a traditional Chinese practice from which anyone could derive health benefits. Cadres and scientists initially supported and even participated in qigong practice. Believed to enhance health and productivity without much capital investment, the practice was expected to produce ideal citizens who did not need health care as the state labored to further develop the market.

The tide of popularity associated with specific masters meant, however, that new figures not necessarily affiliated with the state bureaucracy emerged as powerful entrepreneurs and political players. When noticeable numbers of practitioners started experiencing hallucinations and loss of control over mind and body, this provided an opportune moment to declare such practitioners chaotic and unfit for the new levels of flexibility that participation in a world economy demanded. Lack of productivity and sickness reduced a worker's capacity to create surplus value, hence new forms of postsocialist order were valorized. Although qigong was widely regarded as promoting health, ironically, certain forms could potentially worsen or even bring out new pathologies. Regardless, it was widely accepted as a powerful tool capable of pushing the normative boundaries of institutions and states.

PSYCHIATRY AND ANTHROPOLOGY

Questioning the social norms that define mental illness was an early contribution of anthropologists interested in cultural difference. Edward Sapir, an anthropologist who is best known for his extensive contribution to the study of linguistics, noted in 1932 that "cultural anthropology, if properly understood, has the healthiest of all skepticisms about the validity of the concept 'normal behavior.' It cannot deny the useful tyranny of the normal in a given society but it believes the external form of normal adjustment to be an exceedingly elastic thing" (1985, 514). His essay "Cultural Anthropology and Psychiatry" pointed out that anthropology was "valuable because it is constantly rediscovering the normal" (515) or the means by which categories of human behavior are established. Anthropologists have thus mainly addressed mental illness as a mapping of social values and cultural beliefs that shape the norms and situated knowledges that categorize human behaviors. For instance, the qualities that might make someone a shaman in indigenous or tribal communities so powerful—visions, the ability to communicate with spirits, and other capabilities—could easily be diagnosed as symptoms of schizophrenia in the culture of biomedicine. The study of mental illness from a medical perspective has primarily focused on deviance and abnormality; this places individuals irrevocably in a system of binary and ethnocentric definitions. The anthropological instinct to question the normal has helped to broaden the study of mental illness to include social meanings of madness. By drawing attention to the ways we make boundaries between the normal and the pathological, as Canguilhem (1989) demonstrated in his study of the history of disease and pathology, norms reveal more about social structures and institutions than about the afflicted.

During the mid-twentieth century, two main approaches to culture and psychiatry emerged. In the salvage tradition of ethnomedicine, which documented indigenous medicines and remedies before they disappeared, ethnopsychiatry focused on traditional forms of mental illness and healing (Kluckhorn 1962; Linton 1956). Native American, African, Asian, and other indigenous views of mentality were documented to identify key categories or cultural patterns in a given society. In the medium of ethnographic film, Jean Rouch's controversial 1952 film *Les maîtres fous* vividly juxtaposed immigrant Hauka possession rituals with the legacy of colonial rule. The film argued for the possibility that such indigenous rites helped to recuperate a sense of self and well-being in the rapidly urbanizing African context far more effectively than did treatment in the mental ward. On the other hand, crosscultural psychiatry addressed localized forms of psychiatry and institutions of mental health practices usually in non-Western countries (Marsella and White 1982; Kleinman and Good 1985). Studies from this approach raised a central problem: how to understand within assimilated models of psychiatry illnesses that clearly have cultural dimensions. Kleinman's research in particular has addressed the issue of diagnostic categories most keenly in his concepts of explanatory models and somatization (1980).

Foucault's (1973) analysis of madness in Europe from the end of the sixteenth century to the eighteenth century conceptualized shifts in historical practices and social context as a means to trace civilizational discourses. A compelling part of his analysis was the focus on the asylum as a very specific place in time and space. Medical historians have productively engaged with psychiatry in terms of its social histories and the practices taking place within certain institutions such as Salpêtrière, Bicêtre, and Bethlam (Porter 1987). Such places were transient, because of their eventual closures, their transformations in practice, and, not least, the marginalized inpatients retained there. And yet certain physical structures and social relations of institutions transcend and continue even though the people who pass through them are no longer present.

Another critical contribution by anthropologists to the study of psychiatry has been through in-depth ethnographic documentation within clinics and inpatient wards. Ethnographers based in such clinical contexts thus have multiple roles: to go beyond the dyadic doctor-patient relationship and contextualize medical authority within the social and political ethos of the era; to document structures of health care and their histories; and to locate within these stories the lives of ordinary people. Ethnographic studies within psychiatric institutions over the past two decades have traced the shift from discursive elements of therapy to deinstitutionalization as well as viewing the social contexts of mental illness (Estroff 1981; Rhodes 1991; Scheper-Hughes 1979; Kleinman 1986).

Globalization is not a new notion in this profession, particularly since international congresses and meetings have for decades standardized professional codes of classification for behavior and treatment. What the anthropology of psychiatry has offered to counter such globalizing discourses is a steadfast focus on psychiatric practices through grounded ethnographic accounts of knowledge and power. More recent analyses of such practices have critically compared the uses of global psychiatry to alternative forms of healing for emotional and psychological disorders (Gaines 1992; Sharp 1993).

As biomedicine itself has increasingly become the object of study in medical anthropology, classification categories have been examined as documents that reflect culturally specific ideologies and practices (Young 1997). In their elegant analysis of the power of invisible categories in shaping everyday life, Bowker and Star (1999) show how classifications are important technologies of states and institutions of power. During the twentieth century, "large modern states have found themselves forced into development of complex classification systems to promote their political and economic smooth functioning" (34). Classifications are important forms of political shorthand to achieve social order. In a sense, culture-bound syndromes have the potential to undo globally accepted categories as such conditions point out the importance of differences and the difficulty of cultural translation. If, however, these culturally specific disorders can be folded into a special category of their own, then difference can be contained, and progress can be resumed once more. Thus the recent inclusion of more culture-bound syndromes in the latest DSM-IV, the acknowledged classificatory guide in psychiatry, suggests a wider acceptance among psychiatrists of culture and difference in mental illness.

In the Chinese context, the practice of psychiatry has frequently been shaped by politics. While the former Soviet Union became known for state abuses of "penal psychiatry" where political dissidents were locked up in insane asylums, the forms of politicized psychiatry in China incorporated Maoist theory in treatment, instead. Recent accounts have raised concerns about the punishment of dissidents within the Chinese legal system (Munro 2000). The allegations inevitably draw comparisons to the former Soviet Union, whose psychiatric profession was denounced by world associations for such practices. In response to Munro's characterization of Chinese psychiatry as politically organized, Kleinman and Lee indicate the slippery slope of adopting this view, which does not apply to the majority of general psychiatric practice (2002). Ordinary psychiatrists work hard with families to offer mental health care, especially as it is a precious and limited resource: the number of hospital beds is very small. Moreover, the profession increasingly follows global diagnostic categories.

Forensic psychiatry, which deals with legally insane people who face criminal charges, often operates separately from mainstream psychiatry in both China and the West. Like their counterparts in the West, Chinese police are often the first to encounter mad people on the streets and have to decide whether to bring them to jail or to the mental hospital. Veronica Pearson's (1995) analysis of mental illness, law, and rights in China indicates that while severely retarded individuals are not considered to be fully responsible for their actions, mentally ill people with sufficient self-awareness to control their own actions can be held responsible, although offenders with potential mental illnesses are examined to determine the extent of that responsibility. In cases of serious psychotics who are dangerous but cannot be held responsible for their actions, "there are special hospitals run by the public security bureau," referred to as *an cun* (peace village) hospitals (1995, 36–40).[14] (Another term for these specialized units for the criminally insane is *ankang* [peace and health] hospitals.)

Chinese psychiatry, or psychiatry in any context, is often characterized as repressive. By documenting the transformation of institutions, diagnostic categories, and physicians, I hope to contextualize further the social and cultural components of Chinese psychiatry. In this book I show how psychiatry is intimately involved in the process of state building and modernization through the medicalization of experience. My research inevitably encounters the questions Foucault raised about discipline and governmentality. I take seriously his lifelong project to characterize the generative aspects of institutions in defining subjects. I diverge, however, by also stepping outside the frame of state institutions to draw on social categories that can help redefine the meaning of healing within a psychiatric ward. Anthropology is an intervention that can reframe the understanding of psychiatry as a dynamic process of cultural translation rather than a rigid institution. By including family members and alternative healers in this ethnographic analysis, I hope to show how institutionalization is part of a broader, eclectic range of possibilities and cultural practices.

QIGONG AS ALTERNATIVE MEDICINE

Since its reemergence in post-Mao China, qigong has become a global phenomenon. It has not only transformed official medicine in China but also spread widely throughout Asia, North America, Europe, and even Latin America. In addition, a number of spinoffs or localized versions of breathwork or energy healing have emerged. Why is qigong so prevalent in so many contexts? It could be argued that its popularity is due solely to wider trends of globalization and the travel of immigrant practitioners.

The promise of healing of course has widespread appeal for people in search of health and self-cultivation. Practitioners both inside and outside China often spoke of their dreams of the good life, visions of well-being and liberation from expensive drugs. Their narratives were especially compelling when viewed as responses to the immense changes and uncertainty of the market economy. Rather than remaining in situations of despair marked by uncertainty, distress, or debilitating illness, practitioners opted to counter their somatized disorders actively by seeking healers and participating in healing exercises. Viewing qigong initially through the lens of what is called alternative medicine offers a different vantage point that reveals how passionate and often desperate searches for healing are shared across cultures.

While the majority of my discussion is based on research carried out in China, my exploration of qigong in Japan, Taiwan, and the United States refers to a different politics of location. Though practitioners described a common search for healing and spiritual meaning in each of these places, the configurations of practice and the ways in which popular images of masters spread were significantly different. One framework for reading qigong—as a culturally specific practice with certain histories of significance—was not enough because the phenomenon shifted in dramatic ways to accumulate a transnational following just as I was conducting field research. As an ethnographer of this healing practice, I needed to move among several frameworks to locate meanings and epistemologies in the making as the practitioners themselves did. This ethnography traces the more recent transnational trend in alternative healing where healers, clients, and communities fluidly travel, cross borders, and share economic interests.

Until the late twentieth century, the travel of medical knowledge, technologies, and ideologies across the Pacific has predominately emphasized biomedicine as the key to modernity and national progress. While medical missionaries traveled throughout East Asia to build hospitals and collaborate with local governments, in the United States practitioners of traditional Asian medicine set up herbal shops and clinics within restricted communities for immigrant clientele. Both traditional healing and Western medicine established a presence in other venues, and yet as medical doctors gained preeminence, traditional medical practitioners initially were patronized only by older generations, while newer generations increasingly turned to Western medicine by midcentury. In contrast to an earlier generation of patient-clients, which practiced alternative healing as a nearly invisible community to mainstream medicine, present practitioners are quite visible and operate in a setting where medical pluralism is increasingly accepted.

In this last section, I use the term "alternative" to represent approaches distinct from the sometimes overlapping categories of traditional and complementary medicine. Alternative medicine in the context of late-twentieth-century North America refers to a wide spectrum of health beliefs and healing practices from multiple sources, ranging from traditional Asian systems of medicine and other established systems of healing such as homeopathy, naturopathy, and chiropractic to more new age forms of healing such as aromatherapy and healing with crystals. Traditional medicines such as acupuncture, ayurveda, and indigenous shamanic medicines are cultural systems of knowledge closely tied to specific plants, pharmacopeias, and healing techniques. Though there might be heterodox or pluralistic schools of theory and practice within each system, these forms of traditional medicine are transmitted over many generations either through oral history or textual knowledge. Many traditional medical systems are holistic in that they promote a long-term approach to healing the whole person and their dis-ease rather than isolating and curing just a disease. Holistic medicine is often used interchangeably with alternative medicine, as both emphasize wellness and treatment of the whole person over a specific pathology and the treatment of acute conditions. Perhaps what is most shared among these diverse systems of medical knowledge has been the hegemonic response by biomedical institutions to categorize, contain, or sometimes denounce such systems. The convergence of such vastly different systems under the umbrella category of alternative over several decades reflects the political landscape of medicine in North America.

As an ethnographer of biomedicine, Robert Hahn (1995) identified several characteristics that alternative systems hold in common, such as holistic views of the mind and body, focus on healing the whole person rather than curing disease, and most critically a reliance on alternative ways to treat chronic illness and disease distinct from biomedical forms of treatment. According to Hahn, biomedicine incorporates the notion of "biologically oriented medicine that predominates in Western societies" (1). Many laypersons still refer to such forms of knowledge and practice as Western medicine. Yet, as medical anthropologists such as Margaret Lock (1980) working in non-Western societies have shown, rather than simply being located in Western societies, biomedicine is best described as a medical system that includes global formations and techniques of biopower in the surveillance and production of suitable subjects. Biomedicine has been imported and practiced worldwide for over a century.

Complementary medicine can be viewed as a middle ground in which both biomedical and alternative medical interventions are employed by patients, often those diagnosed with terminal disease or chronic illness. Rather than choosing one system over another, patients take the pragmatic "whatever works" plural approach to treatment. It is now common for patients to undergo radiation and chemotherapy for cancer treatment and then seek holistic alternatives to recover from the extremely toxic and iatrogenic dosages of bio-medicine. The popular demand, relatively low costs, and efficacy of comple-mentary treatments led many insurance companies and health maintenance or-ganizations to qualify certain alternative medical practices as reimbursable expenses in the 1980s. The biomedical establishment has cautiously and reluc-tantly acknowledged the efficacy of medical treatments such as acupuncture and chiropractic, among others, for specific ailments. What follows is an at-tempt to trace the formation of the category of alternative and the eventual commodification of such practice in late capitalism. In doing so, I hope to show how qigong, as an alternative to official forms of medicine, can occupy vastly different positions in China and the United States. State institutions and regulatory structures have immense power to determine the ways in which al-ternative forms of medicine are practiced.

The establishment of alternative and traditional healing practices with for-mally licensed practitioners and clinics did not begin in the United States un-til the 1970s, when hospital costs and inflation began to soar. Clients of vari-ous backgrounds began to seek more effective and less costly forms of treatment. Border crossings to Mexico and Canada for alternative healing were common among chronic patients seeking more affordable health care or treat-ments that were banned by the FDA, such as laetrile or marijuana for cancer. With increasing public exposure in the United States to long-established sys-tems of homeopathy, herbal medicine, acupuncture, and chiropractic in other countries, the networks of practitioners and clientele have gradually coalesced into an alternative healing community set in relief to the biomedical establish-ment. In the last two decades of the twentieth century, alternative and com-plementary medicines captured the popular imagination and reemerged as compelling possibilities beyond mainstream medicine. In spite of technologi-cal advances in biomedicine, the impulse to seek traditional, natural, and epis-temologically different systems of healing to counter lifelong problems with chronic illnesses deemed incurable or terminal diseases has fundamentally re-shaped the picture of medicine in the United States as well as other countries.

The official medical establishment, embodied by the National Institutes of Health (NIH), Centers for Disease Control (CDC), American Medical Asso-ciation (AMA), and Food and Drug Administration (FDA), among others, has long had an uneasy relationship with such healing practices. Following the Flexner report, an influential document on the training of medical profession-als in biomedicine from the 1910s, official reports in the early part of the twen-tieth century referred to alternative practices as "medical sectarianism" or the "medical fringe" and more often dismissed them with pejorative terms such as "quackery" (Reed 1932; Ludmerer 1999). But the willingness of North Americans at the end of the twentieth century to return and try traditional medicines and herbal remedies resulted in the lucrative development and search for new medicines by most major pharmaceutical firms. Such moves to draw consumers follow a thriving herbal industry, which has returned to the limelight with multibillion dollar sales, expenses mostly unreimbursed by health insurance, that nearly outmatched total government spending on biomedicine. In recognition of the immense draw and burgeoning market that alternative healing practices have come to embody, the NIH organized the Office of Alternative Medicine (OAM), more recently renamed the National Center for Complementary and Alternative Medicine (NCCAM), to study the efficacy of many practices. Supporters of alternative medicine agree that official recognition was long overdue, yet observers note that the budget for this office is slight compared to the overall budget of its parent agency.

During the late twentieth century, commodification of alternatives was based on the allure of natural healing and liberation from medications. The passionate desire to heal chronic illnesses or terminal diseases often means that institutional barriers are more porous as the bodies of individuals move among practitioners of different systems of medical knowledge. Biomedicine and alternative medicines are slowly reaching an accommodation. According to Scott Montgomery (1993) there are actually more "shared discourses" or what Jean Langford (1999) has called "mimetic entanglements" between alternative medicine and biomedicine. Popular literature on complementary and alternative medicine has moved from celebratory accounts to more careful scientific reports based on double-blind studies. Mainstream medical journals also include more comparative studies as well as articles on the efficacy of ethnomedicine.[15]

The interest and acceptance of alternative healing as new age practices during the 1990s recalls the enthusiasm of an earlier generation in the 1960s and 1970s, which traveled to India and Nepal on journeys of spirituality and healing. Many holistic practitioners actually participated in such journeys as young adults and went on to train and become licensed in different medical systems. One crucial difference, however, marks the search for healing in this era. Encounters with shamans, curanderos, and other healers in recent decades have taken place not only in faraway exotic lands but also increasingly in one's own local context. The spatial and temporal compression attributed to late capital is expressed in the rapid transfer of ideas. It is not unusual for healers to travel on global lecture circuits, with attendances in the hundreds at each stop. Conventions on a large scale such as the Whole Life Expo, smaller workshops sponsored by health food stores or bookstores, and local chapters of adherents of a particular healer or method have made access to knowledge about different forms of healing vastly more available.

While qigong in the North American context can be understood as an alternative or traditional healing practice, my analysis of this practice in a very different context hopes to offer a more nuanced understanding of the cultural dimensions of medicine. Though healing practices and beliefs may travel quickly, circulate widely, and exist simultaneously in all corners of the world, their historical contexts and political meanings can differ and matter greatly. While traditional Chinese medicine and martial arts have been practiced for over a century in the United States, qigong did not reach the North American public scene until the 1980s. Similar to acupuncture and martial art forms, the practice primarily circulated in Asian immigrant and Asian American communities. Interest gradually developed in other followers after they heard miraculous tales or had firsthand encounters with the masters who began to travel frequently throughout this country. A critical moment of cultural translation that took place in the early nineties further contributed to the prominent place qigong began to occupy in the public eye. In 1993 a special PBS series, *Healing and the Mind*, by Bill Moyers, a well-known journalist, took North Americans on a journey exploring the potential of mind-body medicine that reincorporated hope and self-healing. Moyers (1993) mentioned his own encounters with modern medicine, which were alienating and ineffective in treating, for instance, his father's chronic headaches. The series featured many medical doctors who were equally concerned about the art of healing and whose clinical work and research addressed the mind-body connection. In particular, one episode filmed in China focused on the "the mystery of chi." Viewers who might not have heard of qi or qigong were able to see qigong masters heal individuals with the healing touch of this vital energy. Dr. David Eisenberg, who wrote about qigong in the 1970s in *Encounters with Qi* (Eisenberg and Wright 1985), was included as an interlocutor for the special segment. When Moyers and Eisenberg went to clinics or parks and spoke to qigong masters, American audiences saw demonstrations and heard first-hand narratives about this form of healing.

As an ethnographer of this practice in China and other parts of Asia, I found that many people in the United States had already been exposed to the powers of healing possible in this practice of breathing, deep visualization, and concentrated energetic healing at the hands of a master when I returned to the United States in 1991. Rather than facing quizzical looks or blank stares when I spoke of qigong, I experienced quite the opposite response. Like the people I encountered in China, acquaintances and strangers alike would easily engage in conversation about qigong. Their narratives often addressed the miraculous nature of the practice and entailed exuberant accounts of masters and the hard-to-believe results they produced. Most lay practitioners I have encountered in both countries recount stories of facing chronic problems with allergies, asthma, or eating disorders. Other interviewees have faced even more serious illnesses such as cancer or immune disorders. Their primary motivation for trying qigong was an attitude of "why not?" and a search for something that could fill the gaps between modern medicine and daily struggles with chronic illness or terminal disease. While practitioners of qigong in the United States were initially ethnic Chinese or Asian American, within several years the practice has quickly crossed ethnic and cultural borders. Practitioners from visibly upper-middle-class and professional backgrounds indicate that qigong has been rapidly accepted and enfolded in the alternative healing movement. Today, there is also a thriving market in qi-related products such as the instant qi herbal elixir, the qi watch, and qi videos that target consumers of all backgrounds (Frank 1998).

Just as qigong in North America has fit into the rubric of alternative and traditional medicine, in China the practice also operated as an alternative to state or official systems of health care. Though some hospitals of traditional Chinese medicine offered forms of qigong healing and even held regular qigong outpatient clinics, immense numbers of people practiced qigong individually or in large groups in the parks, on the streets, in work units, or in large gymnasiums. The social life of qigong engendered by its practitioners and by the attention from state media, popular publications, and scientific discourses produced a very different experience over there. What initially began for many as a way of healing a nagging ailment or a search for a healthy lifestyle quickly turned into a social movement that led some state representatives to question the mass appeal of some forms of practice and the masters associated with these forms.

New age practices of holistic healing have an extensive background in Europe and the United States. There is a long-established cultural receptivity to practices such as qigong. It is nearly impossible to address the practice without considering the charismatic leaders who have led such healing movements. In an essay on charismatic movements in the nineteenth and twentieth centuries, including Native American ghost dances, Pentecostal faith healings, and cargo cults, Anthony F. C. Wallace (1961) wrote that such phenomenal followings and practices would not be possible without the critical involvement of dynamic and engaging leaders who can mobilize individuals to act as a social entity or superorganic whole. Even before mass media, charismatic leaders often transformed local groups into large networks of followers. In the present moment of mass communication and consumption, new figures continue to foster desires for communitas and healing via channels of consumption. For instance, in the 1990s Deepak Chopra, guru of the new age movement, regularly brought alternative spiritual practices into the mainstream, commodifying them at the same time. According to a *Newsweek* cover story in 1997, his diversified web of self-help lectures, center services, books, CDs, and supplements together form an enterprise with profits of $15 million annually (Leland and Power 1997). In recent years, some qigong masters have also amassed great followings and assembled enterprises that include healing centers and lecture circuits as well as numerous sites disseminating core philosophies via books, tapes, CDs, and the Internet. Popular healing in such instances exists not simply because of the vast networks generated by such charismatic healers but also because of the commodification of healing knowledge that speaks to ordinary desires to achieve order and balance in complex times.

Such formulations of alternative medicine linked to specific leaders or authority figures raise questions of authenticity. There are no standard bases to evaluate the qualifications of these healers beyond the networks of belief that led to their rapid rise. Any analysis of qigong in China and beyond must thus be mindful of markets in which it has thrived as a popular healing practice. The current celebratory and lucrative embrace of alternative medicines in the United States and other countries often overlooks social histories of translation and usage. For instance, qigong is often included in the category of traditional Chinese medicine rather than understood as having its own history.

Rather than presuming that the practices of breath work, meditation, and healing associated with qigong are uniform in meaning and reception, this ethnography aims to show how cultural translations of medicine and the contexts of healing practices matter greatly. Critically engaged readings of alternative medicine that examine cultural contextualization can counter the overly enthusiastic reception of different medical practices. In this spirit, my findings suggest a less well known side of healing, where too much of a good thing can sometimes become harmful. For some individuals, without proper knowledge and supervision, the practice of qigong could bring bouts of dizziness, indigestion, headaches, dysphoria, anxiety, and even intense pain, among other symptoms.[16] Moreover, as socialized medicine in China has already faded into profit-oriented forms of medicine in a market economy, the influence healers had on patients and the totalizing experiences seekers sometimes found themselves enmeshed in are worthy of discussion and critique.

STRUCTURE OF TEXT

I examine four specific periods relevant to the practice of qigong: expansion, medicalization, transnational circulation, and anticult regulation. The initial interest and widespread expansion of qigong took place in the decade of reforms after Mao (1979–89). In chapter 2, I address how the general public in China became crazy for qigong, gripped by has been referred to as qigong fever, and how eventually some individuals' fervent practices drove them to erratic behaviors. As I have already noted, for a brief period, qigong flourished as a highly charismatic social medicine that eventually became regulated and reclaimed as state medicine. The year I began my field research, however, a new period of medicalization and regulation was commencing. Though the practice of qigong continued to grow and new masters surfaced, from 1989 to 1994 key figures within the scientific, psychiatric, and administrative communities came together to regulate the practice. The post-Mao state's efforts to bottle the genie of mass interest were rather unsuccessful at first. It wasn't until significant numbers of patients emerged in the psychiatric wards that the state managed to contain the popularity of certain masters and forms of qigong. The emergence of the psychiatric category of qigong deviation, the coalescence of the state apparatus, and the introduction of licensing regulations during this short time sought to contain the fever (*jiangwen*) that swept most cities. The ensuing years of 1995–99 seemed quiet in comparison, as the Chinese market went global. With increased participation in the world economy, interest in qigong practice dwindled. This, however, was the moment when qigong went global and new forms of spiritual practice and body cultivation such as falungong emerged. Since 1999, the official stance of the government has been decidedly anticult, with little room even for qigong practitioners. Along with anticorruption trials, much energy has been devoted to the eradication of spiritual groups that are viewed as obstructive to the progress of the nation.

In chapter 3, I discuss the emergence of qigong masters that fanned the quick spread of the practice across China. The paths to becoming a master are quite eclectic. Some masters are reclusive and try to avoid acquiring sectlike followers, while others base their expertise in generations of knowledge and practice. Quite a few proclaim themselves to be masters without having come from any previously known lineages of practice. Though Deng Xiaoping deemphasized the cult of the leader to facilitate transitions of power, masters easily stepped into the limelight and took on the charismatic authority that Mao formerly embodied. Discourses of the superhuman and paranormal circulated, and qigong masters were believed to be capable of all powers. I also address the gender politics of this category, since the majority of masters represented in popular narratives were hypermasculine figures. By contrast, the state campaign to arrest one female master revealed the political cosmology of power in contemporary Chinese politics.

Chapters 4 and 5 examine the psychiatric context and growing management of qigong-related disorders. Chapter 4 addresses the specific phenomenon of qigong deviation, a culture-bound syndrome that emerged in Chinese clinics in the 1990s, first within the clinical setting and then outside the clinic as part of popular discourses. In this disorder, the individual mind and body became unbound; sufferers could lose control over their limbs, sensory perceptions, or bodily functions. Emotional and psychological breakdowns accompanied the loss of bodily control. Further, sensations of being possessed or otherwise controlled by outside entities led to expressions of emotional or physical disorder. Sometimes afflicted individuals experienced terror and fear, but qigong deviation also produced ecstatic mania and feelings of omnipotence and invincibility. Patients' inability to carry out social and political responsibilities became a key concern for family members and state institutions. Somehow, individuals had to be contained and retrained for their proper social roles.

Chapter 5 looks at the contemporary structure of Chinese mental asylums and the practices within hospital inpatient wards and outpatient clinics. This chapter weaves together several narratives and historical strands that led to the institutionalization of psychiatry in twentieth-century China. Many accounts of this process focus on the clinical encounter between doctor and patients, leaving out the role of families and the social experiences of madness. The mundane everyday dramas of caring for an unbalanced family member when one's own resources are depleted has been rarely addressed.

The practice of self-healing through regulating the breath and turning to masters instead of official doctors for help further emphasized the distance between state medical care and personal states of well-being. Indigenous notions of spiritual deviation in qigong practice were increasingly defined and treated by psychiatric means. The order prescribed by the state depended on the notion of the psychiatric hospital as provider of ideal sanity. But such centers only occupied the peripheries of the larger stage that the Chinese socialist state was actively constructing for the Asian Games in 1990. The games were intended to jump-start the economy and reinvigorate morale. In contrast to the stigmatic silence associated with popular images of the mental hospital, the din of the games, promoted as grand spectacle, only intensified attention to the distance between the official ideology enforced by martial law and personal experiences of disruption. While official gestures of openness to the world and return to social stability were emphasized, such staged messages meant little to those who no longer considered themselves to be in the audience any longer.

The state apparatus's move to medicalize qigong and contain the popularity of certain masters involved a gradual mobilization of official media, bureaucrats, health officials, and scientists. Chapter 6 addresses the critical role of scientists and scientific discourse in cleansing the ranks of practitioners by pathologizing certain forms. In the ensuing dichotomization of "real" science from pseudoscience, masters were expected to conform to new rules of practice such as becoming licensed to join the state system or risk being viewed as having "false" powers. Ultimately, the regulation of qigong secularized many forms, so that followers either adapted or went underground to continue their practices. Another result was the transnational travel of masters to venues outside mainland China. As few masters dared practice without licenses and even fewer held popular performances, qigong fever appeared to have subsided or even disappeared by the mid-1990s when China returned to full participation in the global market economy.

Chapter 7 addresses the flow of masters and formations of qigong communities in Taiwan, Japan, and the United States. Like practitioners within the PRC, most people were drawn to the pursuit by fantastic stories of the power of qigong masters or eyewitness accounts of healing. Charismatic healers who claimed to be able to heal any disorder with qigong traveled widely, appealing to those in search of answers to chronic pain and illness. New technologies such as the Internet were also incorporated to facilitate broader means of outreach and communication for practitioners. The development of qigong groups unbound by state regulations or spatial and temporal factors led to the proliferation of several organizations of new masters. One group in particular, the Falungong organization, which eclectically incorporated qigong exercises with self-cultivation, religious iconography, and new age spiritualism, became infamous for its overt political protest on the eve of the fiftieth anniversary of the PRC and the tenth anniversary of Tiananmen demonstrations. The subsequent response of the body politic synonymous with the state evoked earlier crackdowns on "false" and "unscientific" qigong at the beginning of the decade. By placing itself on the stage the state was meant to occupy, Falungong was quickly established as a political threat and made into an example of anti-science and *mixin* (superstition), the very elements that Chinese socialism has been devoted to eradicating in its fifty years of history.

Just as the Chinese government wished to create boundaries of order, individual practices of spiritualism offered the possibility of transcending such containment. The shared discourses on order and yet contradiction of these divergent strategies for attaining stability reveal how the late socialist state has operated incongruently in response to the needs of individuals.[17] For the purpose of this analysis, the contemporary Chinese state will be considered not only as a monolithic bureaucracy but also as an entity composed of individuals with fluid identities that can at times contradict the system. Such a perspective acknowledges the formal hegemonic structures of power as well as the intentions, desires, and actions of individuals that are interwoven into the fabric of a state corpus. My intent is to bring into focus the negotiations that ordinary people and officials face in various arenas, revealing multiple and even contradictory roles in public and private realms. I remain most compelled by the sincere desires of lay practitioners who were just hoping for some answers to their somatic disorders.

The continued appeal of qigong and new spiritual practices reveals how powerful and pervasive Chinese traditions of healing and inner body cultivation can be. Self-cultivation and group practice provide the foundations for forging communal notions of identity that can transcend socialist formations of *hukou* (registered permanent residence) or *danwei* (work unit) that are the fundamental units of the state (Lu and Perry 1997). Yet, even with unruly masters and the potential for subversive actions, the Chinese body politic continues to promote qigong as an efficient healing practice, primarily because it is uniquely Chinese and promotes an important element of state identity. As one state bureaucrat remarked in interview, "Qigong is a treasure-house of China, and we need to protect it from unsavory characters who use it to sell themselves. All the Japanese and westerners come here to learn about qigong because they can't find anything comparable to heal themselves." Qigong remains popular because of the prevalence of long-term or chronic illnesses in many cultures. The practice offers individuals the sensual pleasure of transforming the body through healing. As the Greek philosopher of medicine Galen observed, "All medicine is politics." Whether in a socialist or late capitalist context, healing is very much a part of everyday life and often entails a political act of imagining and pursuing alternatives.

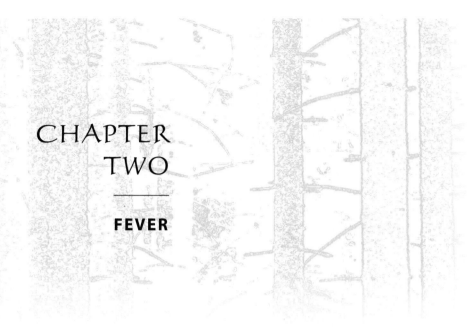

CHAPTER TWO

FEVER

ON AN OVERNIGHT TRAIN journey from Shanghai to Beijing during the spring of 1990, I listened to a broadcast of two comedians engaged in quick banter.[1] One comedian began by asking the other performer whether he believed in qigong. His colleague began to recount the amazing deeds of a master who could heal anything, including his baldness, at which the taped audience began to laugh. After the ten-minute sketch moved on to a satire of regional accents and puns, passengers in the hard sleeper section began to discuss whether qigong really could live up to all the claims made by masters. A thin bespectacled man in a beige woolen vest listened as a fellow passenger, an older male in his sixties, extolled the virtues of a master he was planning to see in Beijing. The first man responded with questions and anecdotes of his own encounters with qigong. Fueled by innumerable cups of tea and cigarettes, the conversation lasted into the night as onlookers also contributed remarks on the subject. By the time the train began to roll into Beijing station, several of the passengers had exchanged name cards or addresses and even agreed to meet at a local park. It was clear that qigong had arrived long before as a hot topic.

The widespread expansion of qigong began in the decade of reform after Mao (1979–1989), coinciding with the state's effort to embrace a market economy. This period has been referred to by many Chinese as qigong *re* (fever). During the Maoist years mass propaganda, disseminated via work units, village cadres, and neighborhood grannies, helped to maintain rigid boundaries of thought and behavior for the general population. As post-Mao reforms shifted to economic revitalization, new possibilities for personal agency and embodiment also emerged. This chapter examines how qigong fever presented a potential disruption to the Chinese body politic on the fast track to modernization. I also explore how it was a specific response to the stresses of economic and social change.

What could inspire so many people to become interested or believe in qigong? In what follows, I track the development of qigong in three contexts. Emile Durkheim's (1986) views of the social forces that organize and motivate people, what he called the superorganic, argue powerfully for an understanding of collective behavior.[2] Max Weber (1994) characterized the convergence of individuals' moral and economic behavior as a collective ethos. Social historians have illuminated how overwhelmingly popular desires for tulips or sightings of religious figures had widespread consequences.*Memoirs of Extraordinary Popular Delusions*, an 1853 study of popular movements by Charles Mackay, documented moments when beliefs promoted by charismatics or shared by groups rapidly progressed into frenzied behaviors that ultimately led to the collapse of the existing symbolic and material world: "In reading the history of nations, we find that, like individuals, they have their whims and their peculiarities; their seasons of excitement and recklessness, when they care not what they do. We find that whole communities suddenly fix their minds upon one object, and go mad in its pursuit; that millions of people become simultaneously impressed with one delusion, and run after it, till their attention is caught by some new folly more captivating than the first" (1980, xvii). Indeed, the parallels can be found everywhere. Melanesian cargo cults during the nineteenth century are read by scholars as local responses to cultural contact. These cults ostensibly focused on European material goods but were also enmeshed in wider webs of popular activities characterized as "nativistic," "messianic," or "millenarian" (Burridge 1995; Cochrane 1970). Alison Winter's compelling social history of mesmerism reveals how, like qigong, the belief in magnetism accumulated both mystical as well as scientific meanings. The spread of mesmerism, the belief in magnetic healing powers, throughout eighteenth- and nineteenth-century Europe took hold in Victorian Britain in such a way that it transformed existing discourses of medicine, science, and religion. Philip Kuhn's (1990) analysis of epidemic fears about sorcery in imperial China during 1768 traces how concerns about soul stealing could travel and transform the worldviews of vast numbers of individuals, including official bureaucrats. Desires for health and fears about sorcery are at the center of many fads, and such social phenomena are not limited to the distant past. During the years of the Cultural Revolution, many Chinese faced with food shortages engaged in a number of health fads purported to enhance vitality, among them, rooster blood infusions (1969–70), drinking cold water (1972–73), and *shrai shou* (vigorous hand movements, 1975–76).[3] Even in the 1990s iconic images of Chairman Mao were prominently hung in Chinese cabs and some rural households to bring good fortune.

The 1990s saw other fads or popular pursuits, such as stock market fever and even culture fever (Hertz 1998). Jing Wang (1996) notes that this was a period when writers and other intellectuals, in salons and in journals, engaged in intense debate over history, national identity, and individuality.[4] As cultural brokers in different media, Chinese filmmakers, artists, and musicians were gaining recognition from foreign audiences and patrons for their creative work. For urban residents of all backgrounds, the development of free markets meant more access to material items as well as new ideas. Shifts in political culture to embrace entrepreneurialism and market lifestyles greatly transformed views of leisure time and personal space. As market reforms reconfigured city life, the desire to inject personal meaning into such realms was even more pervasive. The pursuit of personal interests and private spheres of meaning was accompanied by temporal and spatial transformations both at home and in very public spaces. In parks, in addition to participating in taiji and qigong group practice, people openly danced to disco music and Western waltzes formerly dismissed as decadent.

Relaxed controls and the privatization of publishing facilitated the social emergence of qigong masters as public figures, whose books, tapes, lectures, and public demonstrations gained rapt audiences. Throughout China, fervent discussions about the power of qigong took place wherever the opportunity arose. The immense popularity of masters and highly visible practices taking place throughout China ignited conversations and debates about the miracles of qigong among strangers, acquaintances, and family members. In a sense, qigong reframed the very boundaries of public and private spheres, opening different possibilities for the organization of daily life in time and space.

Rather than coordination with state-imposed spatial and political order, qigong practitioners sought personal balance and self-cultivation through attention to healing practices. For instance, *bigu*, the Daoist practice of fasting and meditation, became quite fashionable, especially when qigong masters advocated this as a means of purging illness and achieving spiritual purification to reach higher levels of healing. Ms. Jin, an accountant in her forties who frequented Purple Bamboo Park, claimed to have not eaten for weeks, even months, energized solely with special water and meditation. Family members who did not understand or support such practices were deeply disturbed by the sight of loved ones undergoing rapid physical and mental transformations. Mrs. Guo, a woman in her sixties, spoke passionately, tears in her eyes, when a casual conversation turned to bigu. "How can my son survive if he doesn't eat grains? I've seen him shrink before my eyes." Her son, an academic in his forties, believed that his practice would enhance his qigong abilities further. "I used to have headaches and suffer from neurasthenia. The drugs, herbs, and acupuncture didn't work. Now I'm free of all that. I feel tremendous after reversing my life course." Many practitioners who underwent the process of purification spoke of feeling energized and enlightened afterward. Such forms of self-cultivation were not taken up merely because so many were promoting the fad; they also achieved popularity as effective means to attain the fitness necessary to withstand the disruption the whole society was undergoing.

MANAGING CHAOS

The feverish interest in qigong can also be contextualized in terms of the dual themes of chaos and order in Chinese culture. The notion of disorder (*luan*) is a prevalent theme in Chinese philosophy and Daoist spiritual beliefs. It has also been a long-term concern in state discourse. Although luan is considered a formative elements in nature and characteristic of humanity, literary descriptions of chaos in twentieth-century China tended to locate it within social and political formations. During the Maoist era, urban centers were considered to be decadent and turbulent places, and rural work was promoted as rehabilitation. I contend that socialism was founded on the platform of social stability as an antidote to the previous century of disorder and disruption.

Even though the four modernizations (industry, agriculture, science and technology, and national defense) were invoked frequently as the primary goal of the post-Maoist state, the Chinese bureaucracy, both past and present, has valued social order even more. The project of socialist modernization was thus a campaign for order, and citizens were expected to conform and embody its ideals. The unifying mentality of the collective in work units and communes was guided by Maoist fervor to attain political and economic independence. The state institutions and ethos forged in the Maoist years became deeply embedded in daily lives by providing and thus determining such necessities as residence, education, health care, work opportunities, and sometimes monthly grain allowances or food bonuses in the post-Mao years.

The drive for modernization has been a concern of the Chinese government throughout different periods. The buildup of a Chinese state apparatus has been justified in terms of the greatly increased needs of the world's largest population, which meant intervention at every level of social integration and personal life (Duara 1988; Shue 1988). In such a system, order emanated from a

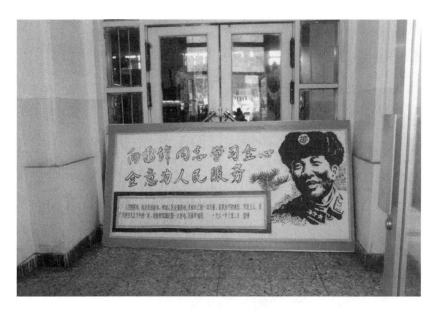

2. Lei Feng poster in department store entrance

central body. While meeting the needs of a population of 1.2 billion was a main concern, the move to prepare citizens to become appropriate subjects was an equal challenge for post-Mao policies (Anagnost 1997). Socialist discourses continue to reverberate with narratives of order and the necessity of maintaining social stability. In the post-Tiananmen period, preschoolers, university students, and all urban residents were urged once again to learn from the example of Lei Feng, a resurrected and reinvented hero who had died nearly thirty years before for the greater good of Communism during the Cultural Revolution. At key sites in state markets, street corners, and schoolyards, posters and banners to "Study from Lei Feng" were used to encourage citizens to cultivate desired socialist traits of selflessness and devotion (see fig. 2).[5]

Post-Mao modernization programs and open-door policies have greatly affected material, social, and emotional life in contemporary China. Rapid urbanization and the embrace of the market economy have brought a dramatic shift from macro policy to micro politics. Spatial and temporal restructuring rely on disciplined bodies for production in a global economy. On factory floors, the micro politics of time management and self-discipline have been directed toward workers, especially women. Lisa Rofel's (1999) ethnography of the impact of Chinese modernity on silk factories documents the state's desire

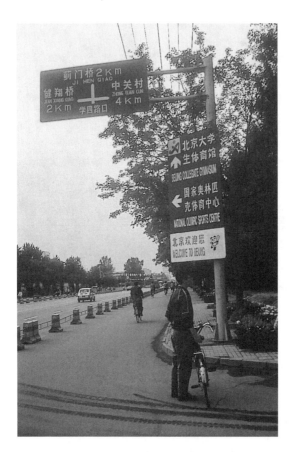

3. New street signs erected in 1990

for well-functioning units and workers. As the micro processes of such change involve spatial and temporal practice, even embedded forms of exchange have also been transformed. Mayfair Yang's (1994) analysis of the *guanxi* system (networks) illustrates how social relationships were reconfigured to fit the contours of contemporary state practices.

The year 1989 was a watershed moment of political change throughout China, Eastern Europe, and the Soviet Union. The post-Mao state was entrenched in an ideological struggle for social order after the tumultuous Tiananmen demonstrations of 1989. Though the student demonstrations and social unrest in China did not unseat the gerontocracy, significant steps were taken to address public sentiments about corruption and access to material goods. The in-

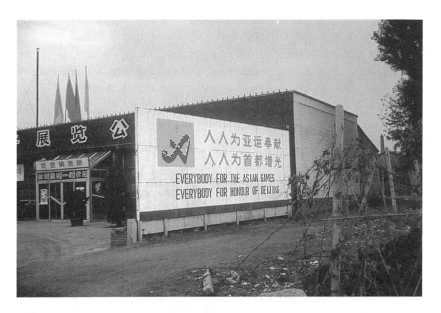

4. Billboard in Haidian district, Beijing, advertising the 1990 Asian Games

sertion of state order took place at several levels. Newer and younger cadres took on more visible leadership roles in both the Communist Party and local municipalities. On an everyday level, the spatial organization of streets and other public sites was employed as a means to establish order and respond to concerns about chaos (see fig. 3).

During the winter of 1990, Beijing residents faced tight restrictions on social gatherings and political expression. Martial law was enforced for over six months, and it was understood that one needed to be discreet when the issue was politics. Life had officially returned to normal, and all citizens were expected to contribute to the success of the Asian Games, the first major international endeavor by the government since the civil unrest of the previous year. Citizens were subjected to a barrage of state propaganda for the coming games in September 1990 (see fig. 4). Great emphasis was placed on cleaning the streets of all major cities and restoring social contentment. During this time, local markets in Beijing bulged with food items, rendering almost indistinguishable the difference between Chinese stores and the Friendship store, which catered to foreign residents and tourists. New street signs in English and romanized pinyin were erected, while new stands for traffic police were installed at every intersection. Instead of the familiar chaos of daily traffic, commuters faced a restrictive order of inconvenient stop signs and citations. Work units, factories, free markets, parks, and especially the streets were the settings for both repair and stepped-up surveillance in the pageantry of socialist modernization. Such steps have been repeated each time China has made a bid for the 2000 and 2008 Olympics.

Postsocialism has been used to describe the transformation of formerly socialist culture, politics, and societies since the disintegration of the Soviet Union and the fall of the Berlin Wall. It is a term rife with contradictions and "confusion," as Verdery (1996, 38) points out in her analysis of postsocialism in Eastern European nations. In China, the term has been used to delineate a period of heightened engagement with market liberalization and state capitalism rather than the end of socialism. Instead of emulating capitalism entirely, the PRC has developed practices closer to what has been increasingly referred to as market socialism or late socialism (see Zhang 2001). Even in a seemingly celebratory moment for the market forces of privatization, socialism lives on—not just in nostalgic memories of Mao but especially in state institutions and the practices of bureaucrats who try to affirm the promises made at midcentury that China would "stand on her own two feet."[6] Recent moves by the state government have been intimately linked with ongoing state desires to participate in a global economy.

When I began my field research during the winter of 1990, many colleagues and friends warned me that the streets were dangerous places where anything could happen. The narratives about chaos on the street and in daily life that I heard from patients and family members began to resonate with earlier tales about the Cultural Revolution. It is important to acknowledge, however, that social discourses about chaos sparked by the Tiananmen demonstrations and enduring throughout the 1990s wane in comparison to the extensive and deeper ruptures of the Cultural Revolution. Though the unrest leading up to June 4, 1989, involved intense political demonstrations in the streets of Beijing and other cities, the chaos attributed to such events cannot match the longer-lived social upheaval, displacements, and state violence that took place during the years of the Cultural Revolution that have affected several generations. This period remains the subject of numerous autobiographies, novels, narrative films, and documentaries in what has come to be referred to as "wounded literature" (Barmé and Minford 1988).

During the 1990s the Chinese government continued to reposition itself in the world economy, and both official media and private citizens voiced feelings of disruption and uncertainty. China participated in the global market as a major producer and consumer of goods, becoming the second-largest domestic economy in the world. A shift from the "iron rice bowl" of socialist institutions

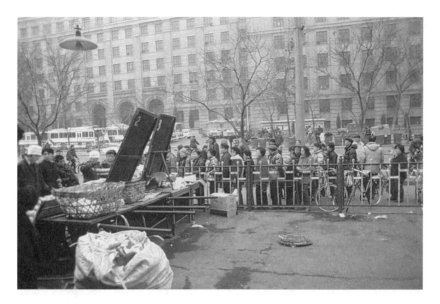

5. Beijing residents waiting at state-run market

to a great sea of opportunities (*xia hai*) has accompanied the vast changes in material and everyday life (see figs. 5 and 6). Despite robust exports and access to new goods and job opportunities, the domestic economy has produced not only nouveau riches but also vastly poorer individuals no longer protected by the familiar net of state welfare and services. The songs of Huxi, a short-lived rock-and-roll band of this time whose name could be translated as "breathing," often invoked the chaotic elements of urban life and feelings of uncertainty about the future.

Ambitious state plans to expand urban spaces, such as the transformations of townships into new cities as well as the continued metropolitan expansion into nearby villages, have literally brought the city to the countryside. The clearing of old buildings, alleyways, and markets for new high-rise office spaces, shopping malls, and private residences has meant a repositioning of the very markers of urban space by which city dwellers used to navigate. The hospital in Beijing where I conducted my field research was demolished, and a new facility erected at a more visible corner of a major intersection.

Recent state campaigns that openly battle corruption, unofficial organizations or networks, and *liumang* (hooligans) have raised the specter of disorder not only at state-level politics but also in everyday life. The dizzying shifts in material and social life in pursuit of capital seem to enhance the disjunctures

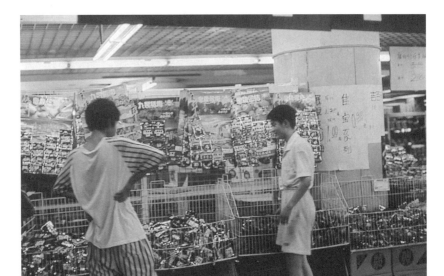

6. A new hypermarket on the top floor of a department store

that were also keenly felt in the 1980s when the post-Mao economy was not yet a critical player in the global economic order. Despite the insertion of the state in daily life at different times and in varying intensities, pursuits and moments of leisure did not have to be tied to the rhythms of the state. As the rapid rise of interest in qigong demonstrated, it was possible to seek alternatives to the daily rhythms of life in Chinese socialism. Qigong was promoted and sought as an antidote to state-induced chaos. Both bureaucrats and ordinary people shared similar desires for order and predictability, yet the means by which this ideal would be achieved were quite different, leading to divergent and even contesting possibilities.

MARKET MEDICINE

The momentous changes in the health care system encouraged the pursuit of more accessible forms of medicine. I have suggested so far two possible explanations for the popularity of qigong: the sway of collective behavior and the desire for order in the face of social chaos. However, I believe that the most compelling reason for the sudden rise in qigong was the special fit for individuals on the move in a dramatically changing economy and health care system. As with other state enterprises that were not turning a profit and even hemorrhaging money, the widely celebrated health care system was gradually restructured into a fee-for-service system during the 1990s (Hsiao 1995; Kahn 1998; Wong and Chiu 1998; Ho 1995; Hesketh and Zhu 1997; Smith 1998; Wu 1997).

Hospitals did not entirely shut down in this restructuring, but services that were once free were increasingly used to generate income for medical institutions that previously had relied entirely on state funding. Drug prescriptions, sonograms, and other lab procedures were some of the services for which patients were now expected to pay for out of pocket rather than be reimbursed through their work unit insurance programs. Such services became vast income generators for hospitals (Lee 1999). The shift to private payment in urban clinics and hospitals reflected the policies that rural health care had been following for nearly a decade. Rather than being reimbursed for their full medical expenses, urban patients were expected to pay any hospital fees up front before services were rendered, just as rural township dwellers and agricultural workers had been expected to do.

Public health literature offers a clear picture of the transition in health care policy. In the early years of socialist medicine, campaigns dedicated to the eradication of pests, improved sanitation, and increased access to health care led to dramatic epidemiological changes (Sidel and Sidel 1973). Infant mortality fell dramatically, as did mortality rates from infectious diseases. The number of health care workers in rural populations increased, and more practitioners were trained in state schools. Yet even with such tremendous improvements, there remained vital gaps between health care in rural areas and urban centers. Over the past fifteen years of "uncoordinated policies," however, health care provisions has devolved from state centralization to the provinces and counties (Hsiao 1995, 1047). While this move would seem to allow for more local autonomy, long-standing regional inequalities have been heightened instead. As the fee-for-service system has been widely adopted, in which new financing and pricing structures are based on user fees, the burden of health care has shifted to patients and their families. The impact of such policies and "increasing inequity and inefficiency" (Hsiao 1995, 1048) can be seen in the serious rise in infant mortality and lack of coverage for basic health care. Infant mortality gradually rose from 34.7 per 1000 in 1981 to 37 per 1000 in 1992. A further dramatic increase took place during the 1990s: the United Nations Children's Fund estimated that the figure rose to 52 per 1000 in the year 2000, an increase of 41 percent in just eight years (Dwyer 2001).

Rural communities have historically had less access to health care despite the heroic interventions of barefoot doctors. In 1975 85 percent of rural dwellers had primary health care coverage. Just over two decades later, in 1997, only 10 percent of rural communities were covered (Carrin et al. 1999; Bloom and Gu 1997). According to a different study on the decline in health insurance, in 1981 less than one-third of the whole population—29 percent—had no health coverage. This figure has more than doubled, to 79 percent (of which 64 percent are rural and 15 percent are urban) (Hsiao and Liu 1996). The number of hospital beds remains the same; however, there are still far fewer than in Japan and the United States (Wu 1997). Gender inequalities have also deepened during the shift to market medicine. Women are less likely to seek professional treatment than males, and young sons receive first priority. Rural Chinese women in particular face extensive inequality and structural violence, with the highest reported suicide rates in the world (Phillips, Liu, and Zhang 1999). The AIDS pandemic has recently been acknowledged as a public health concern. The United Nations estimated in 2001 that over 600,000 people were living with HIV/AIDS in mainland China, with recent infections mainly from unsterilized needles and contaminated blood banks (Lederer 2001).

Deep concern about the disintegration of the existing medical system accompanied the increased popularity of qigong as an alternative form of healing. Biomedical clinics and hospitals in China during the post-Mao era were usually crowded, considered a last resort. Instead, many people relied on herbal remedies, special foods, or tonics, often prepared by family members, before seeking medical advice. It was not uncommon for relatives or friends to share prescribed medications if they thought they were experiencing similar symptoms. Qigong fit easily within this tradition of self-medication and self-sufficiency in healing. Moreover, most practitioners believed that qigong could cure *any* illness or ailment. Part of its appeal was the notion of that regular practice could lead to good health and even superhuman abilities. As examples of the body fantastic, masters demonstrated how the body could become an instrument forged by mind and body together to withstand pain and even heal others. For instance, a young male factory worker once described how qigong allowed him to be more productive and alert even with less sleep than usual.

The broad-based appeal of qigong in the post-Mao era, accompanied by the explosion of mystical movements, arose for several reasons. The motivation most often cited to me by practitioners and masters alike was the desire of individuals to heal themselves rather than rely on continually ingesting numerous medications, whether biomedical prescriptions or traditional Chinese herbs, each day. Whether suffering from chronic pain, injury, or disease, many afflicted sought qigong for initial relief and eventual transformation of their health status from incurable to healed. Especially for somatized complaints or congenital defects, qigong offer a cheaper alternative to the systems of Western medicine and traditional Chinese medicine produced immediate changes. Anyone could buy a book on qigong or go to the parks to take up the practice. Novices could quickly sense the differences in their bodies and experience the movement of qi.

Feeling the body, visualizing internal landscapes, and talking about intimate processes of the body were part of the daily ritual in breathing exercises. Mr. Wang, a retired steel worker in his seventies, took up the practice for his arthritis and rheumatism, which had plagued him for decades. Younger practitioners in their thirties and forties took up the practice to feel energetic and ready for long days at work. As Mr. Zhang, one of the practitioners whom I saw on a daily basis in Tiantan Park, told me, "You see, this way we don't become dependent on drinking cups of coffee every morning like Americans do. If one practices qigong everyday, he or she can be rejuvenated naturally without the aid of stimulants." Qigong was believed to be fast, effective, and inexpensive compared to daily prescriptions. Elderly practitioners in their eighties would often dance circles around me to express the freedom they felt from this change in their daily regimen. Another important reason had to do with the impressive healing powers of charismatic masters, who were believed to be capable of healing most disorders.

Qigong facilitated the shift to market medicine. Promoted by both the state and entrepreneurial masters, qigong fit well with people's desires for better health and less costly prescriptions. Though it could be argued that the pursuit of health has always been integral to Chinese culture, the present moment of vast social and economic changes necessitates an even greater need for healthy bodies. Compared to costly and time-consuming visits to clinics or tradition healers, practitioners found qigong more convenient, inexpensive, and enjoyable. It decreased stresses and anxieties and was believed to improve sensations and energy levels immediately. Moreover, though it could be argued that the pursuit of health has always been integral to Chinese culture, vast social and economic changes necessitated an even greater need for healthy bodies. During the 1980s *suzhi*, the qualities of a people or population who embody a nation, emerged as critical to state projects of modernization. Ann Anagnost has shown that both official and popular discourses of suzhi narrated the lack of culture (*wenhua*) and civilization (*wenming*) possessed by certain overly reproductive bodies that did not function as the productive subjects needed for the modern state (1997, 119).

Medical anthropology provides a powerful lens on the human condition and the lived effects of disruption brought by illness and disease. Analyzing health care policy in particular offers insight into the anxieties and desires of people facing change introduced by market reform. The shift to market medicine deepened already long-standing concerns about health and access to health care. Critically examining affliction and suffering within the larger context of a medical system reveals how much medicine is a reflection of the body politic. Illness narratives, deeply personal histories and stories about the meanings of sickness and disease, provide ways to understand the gravitas of these experiences. Within medical anthropology and biomedicine, these narratives have become important tools to contextualize personal and social meanings in medicine as a window onto culture itself.

In his ethnographic studies of Chinese psychiatry and culture, Arthur Kleinman (1986) notes that "the study of somatization suggests that the body can be a vehicle for experiencing, interpreting, and communicating about emotion and social issues that the person's experience, interpretation, and expression of bodily functions is negotiated in interpersonal relations. Somatic idioms of distress also indicate that in some nontrivial sense the body feels and expresses social problems" (194). Similarly, Robert Hahn points out that sickness refers to "unwanted conditions of self" and as such narratives can be a useful tool in medical anthropology to reveal the intimate and complex relationship among medicine, self, and culture (1995, 22).

Illness narratives continue to be a common social form of discourse in twenty-first-century China. A transformation in narrative content occurred in my interviews with qigong practitioners. All talked about the search for relief as the primary motivation for practice. In that search, the stories of suffering dramatically shifted to journeys of healing. Nearly all the practitioners I interviewed cited health reasons for taking up qigong. Instead of remaining helpless with neurasthenia or terminal diseases, many people took up the practice as an active way to combat the symptoms of chronic illness and somatized distress. Rather than conceiving of healing narratives as oppositional to illness narratives, I suggest that they are part of a continuum. In his analysis of healing, Robert Hahn indicates three related but distinct stages: the remedy (or cure of sickness), rehabilitation (the compensation for loss of health), and palliation (the mitigation of suffering) (1995, 22). Healing narratives describe the continued journey taken by individuals on the road to recuperation. Such a transformation from passive patient to engaged agent in healing is crucial to rethinking how stories of illness and healing shape the world. The journeys toward healing encompass both personal and political spheres.

The practice of qigong in this context revealed desires for affordable medicine and personal meaning while living with intense population pressure and rapid urbanization. Qigong provided a cheap and accessible means of healing in a growing market economy. In certain respects, state agencies tolerated and even encouraged popular interest. In what follows, I outline the contexts in which lay practitioners, scientists, and even officials might initially encounter and eventually pursue the healing art with great passion. Qigong was simultaneously located in three different but overlapping realms: social venues of practice such as parks and courtyards, publishing houses and state media, and the scientific community. The tenor of discussions about qigong in each arena were quite distinct and together contributed to the overwhelming popularity of this practice compared to other forms of healing such as taiji. Though taiji was also a healing exercise that involved the movement of qi through slow meditative steps, it did not generate the widespread and charismatic followers that qigong did. By contrast, the powerful sensations and often immediate transformations of qigong were similar to spiritual conversion. Such experiences sparked the urban imagination and spread feverishly.

BREATHING SPACES

Mornings in most Chinese cities start early. By 5 A.M. street sweepers are on major roads and bypasses, enveloped by large dust clouds as they sweep by hand. Their faces are mostly covered by white gauze masks looped over their ears. Peddlers recycling old plastic containers or bottles move highly stacked mounds of these items on bicycle flats. Giant trucks full of industrial equipment or produce rumble through town. In local neighborhoods, hawkers might ring chimes or chant in local dialect to announce their services or wares. The gates of most major urban parks open, and by 5:30 A.M. small groups of regular visitors with monthly passes are already warming up for their morning exercises (see figs. 7 and 8).

Mr. Yang was an energetic retiree in his eighties who frequently walked around Jin Shan (Coal Hill) Park behind the Forbidden City. On his daily jaunts, he was heartily greeted by other park regulars as he passed. On my second visit to the park, he circled around me twice, and on the third lap he paused to watch me observe practitioners. Mr. Yang warmly invited me to walk around with him as he pointed out the different social groups that were present. As we reached the northern end where the trees were denser and more private, he pointed out a group that met specifically for group healing sessions. Occasionally a master would appear, and long lines would form quickly as she or he would assess each individual's qi or give off healing energies.

Different parks had different groups of practitioners. Though on weekdays I regularly visited a park on my way to the hospital, on weekends I went to the former Temple of Heaven (Tiantan) as this was a very popular site for practice. One early winter dawn I observed about twenty practitioners at the stone

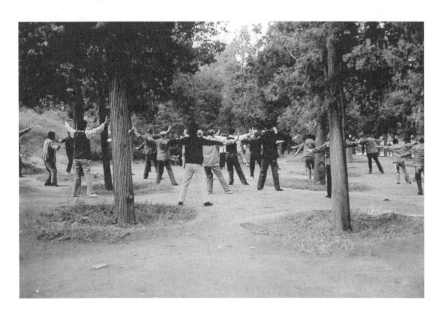

7. Taiji practioners in a Beijing park in a group formation

altar in various states of qi meditation. Some sat in the lotus position, while others stood to concentrate on their breathing or lay on the stone in trances. Nearby, nearly fifty other practitioners danced beneath trees or consulted with each other on the best forms of practice, masters, and daily regimens. Some stood directly in front of particular trees and stepped backward and forward with scooping motions of the arms as if to draw the very essence of the tree into their bodies. Occasionally, deep primal sounds penetrated the morning stillness. A few individuals communicated by speaking in tongues. They all appeared to be ordinary people whom one might encounter throughout the day: store attendants, street sweepers, free market merchants, students, nannies. Qigong practitioners were visibly situated in public parks. Yet their alternative states of consciousness implied a withdrawal from the confines of city and the state. The forms of qigong practice I witnessed were quite different from those I observed in the first park I visited. I soon realized that there were quite diverse forms of qigong practice with very different forms of social spaces and engagement.

The desire to socialize informally with others was also a motivation to participate and take up qigong. One group of lively and vivacious practitioners, all women ranging from fifty to seventy years old, mostly retired, called them-

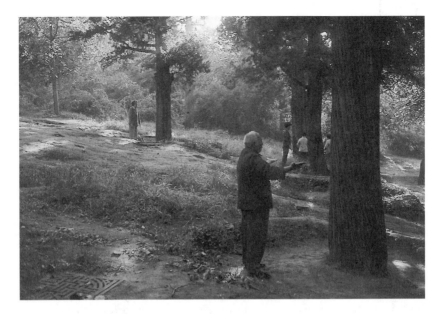

8. Qigong practitioners on other side of same park

selves the thirteen sisters (*shisan jiemen*). The informal group was bound by friendship over two decades and common interests. The majority of them met each weekday morning from 5:30 to 7:30 A.M. to exercise and socialize. Many would banter together before and after practice. Some would arrive when the park gates opened at 6:00 A.M. to reserve their favorite spot by hanging plastic bags or clothes on nearby trees. When one of the sisters, Mrs. Liu, experienced severe headaches and chronic exhaustion, she turned to qigong. On the morning of my visit she showed me her monthly park pass, which had a photo of an older version of herself. "You see, this is what I looked like when I was in pain. I tried all sorts of prescriptions and herbal medicines, but none of them worked. I couldn't go to work if I had a bad day or if it got bad at work; I just had to put my head down." One of the other sisters commented on her improved condition, "Sister Liu looks much younger now, doesn't she? Her color is much better, and she's teaching us her beauty secrets now." They then returned to their trancelike form of qigong, which looked like a cross between taiji and modern dance. Mrs. Liu's healing narrative resembled countless stories from other practitioners. Qigong healing had a redemptive quality that spread quickly in one's social network and beyond.

Trees were integral to certain forms of qigong practice. Many practitioners chose to practice directly in front of specific trees or underneath groves in a quiet park corner. In my first lesson in *yijinjing* (muscle-tendon–changing qigong), Master Wang pointed at a building across the street, stating, "See that? This is what your body is like." He then spread his arms outward under the pine tree that swayed in the slight breeze and fluidly emulated its slight movement. "You need to make your body more pliable and move with the wind as this tree does." Trees not only are a natural symbol for longevity and fruitfulness but also help to provide a sense of place and meaningful practice. According to Laura Rival, "Trees are meaningful not only for what they represent, but also in themselves, as sources of actual and sensual involvement with the world" (1998, 17). In Chinese temples, certain trees are cultivated for their form and longevity. Throughout many parks and former imperial landmarks, trees that have lasted longer than several dynasties are labeled with small plaques. In the homes of urban artists and intellectuals, smaller trees may be carefully cultivated. A grandmother once pointed to a bonsai tree that she had acquired nearly four decades before when her son was born.

Chinese cities in the late twentieth century became ideal settings for the practice and transmission of qigong. How could self-healing practices usually associated with temples nested in hidden mountains become situated in urban townships and metropolitan centers? The shift indicates how qigong was not solely a traditional practice but was also well suited to urban life. Qigong quite literally involved breathing, but such practices transformed people and spaces in very extraordinary ways. In breathing, either in unison with others or alone underneath trees, certain spaces of experience and belonging were generated. The natural and social landscapes offered different types of breathing spaces and relief. The dissemination of information through printed matter and state media facilitated the rapid transfer of knowledge, while social networks provided plenty of anecdotal information. Rather than having dichotomous or oppositional relations with the state, qigong healing often occupied simultaneously spaces created by the state.

Qigong appealed to many laypeople's deep-seated cultural beliefs about health and illness. Mrs. Wu, a food processing factory worker in her sixties, vividly described what drew her to qigong: "Every morning you see people in the parks doing taiji, dancing, or exercising. Qigong fits here because it's Chinese and the movements fit our bodies. I suffer from so many illnesses, and qigong has made me better." Certain forms were viewed as especially appropriate for Chinese ailments such as *shenjing shuairuo* (neurasthenia). Many sufferers took up breathing exercises as an effective means to deal with anxiety or trauma. Though practitioners over the age of sixty were more prevalent in my study, qigong was attractive even to younger people in their twenties. Students in universities who practiced qi cultivation described having renewed energy for their studies.

People to whom I spoke frequently cited how state leaders themselves sought masters for their illnesses, thereby endorsing the practice. Teacher Ding, a regular practitioner in Jin Shan Park put it this way: "Everyone knows that the state leaders wouldn't live so long or so well without the help of the best medical advisers. But the qigong masters provide even more help than traditional medicine. If qigong is good enough for them, it's good enough for *laobaixing* [ordinary people]." Mr. Gao, an architect in his forties, talked about the role that qigong played in his life: "We need to have a personal life in addition to our official life." Taking my pen and notebook, he drew the character *gong* (public), which looks like a capital letter *I*. "See, even this word has two planes to form it. The personal plane is the foundation, while the public plane relies on this. As modern people we need both levels in our life to gain meaning. Without the personal we would just be machines."

The social context of the popular emphasis on healing and self-cultivation made it possible for individuals to meet with other practitioners in times and places that emphasized the rhythms of the body and nature. In addition to demonstrations before large audiences in gymnasiums, practice in public parks allowed for daily informal contact with acquaintances and new members. Participants commented on the ease with which they engaged in conversation or practice: a sense of communitas emerged. Like cafés in nineteenth-century France, the parks as well as other areas where qigong was practiced were key sites of social life for people from all walks of life (Haine 1996).

Institutions and individuals alike operated with ambiguous notions of health and illness. Hospitals, work units, and individuals all accommodated multiple identities that simultaneously embraced public roles and personal meanings in their everyday life. Institutions and work units were the sites of official and unofficial activities, just as individuals assumed many roles throughout the day. Health care workers could be both medical practitioners as well as followers of alternative healing themselves. Occupying the same space was not initially problematic.

The urban socialist landscape continued to be simultaneously transformed by state policies and popular healing practices. As political study was revitalized in universities and key work units to generate social and economic order, the practice of deep-breathing exercises and healing with qigong was never more popular. On campus grounds and at workplaces, qigong masters lectured and demonstrated their powers to students, workers, and even cadres. Arenas became prominent sites where qigong masters demonstrated their powers of healing and raw energy. Dramatic street performances focused on the physical capabilities and external powers of a single master. As in the prerevolutionary China depicted in the San Mao cartoons reproduced in chapter 1, itinerant masters attracted large crowds, which quickly dispersed if necessary. The mass qigong sessions led by more prominent qigong masters in stadiums and elsewhere were impressive not only for the exploits they featured but also for the fact that they could command the attention of hundreds of onlookers, skeptics as well as believers, for hours on end. Huge concrete gymnasiums once filled with avid soccer or volleyball fans were jammed to capacity with thousands of devoted qigong fans and chronically ill or curious individuals seeking the powers of charismatic masters. Not since the Cultural Revolution had spectators occupied these arenas to capacity with such passionate fervor. While initially only dozens of individuals might have visibly emotional responses to a master's lecture, eventually the whole arena would be filled with openly sobbing faces and bodies responding to the qi energy being transmitted. Individuals could be seen writhing on the ground, running up and down aisles, making uncharacteristic body movements, or sitting alone in trances, swaying slightly from side to side. Such scenes often reminded me of evangelical services and even rock concerts, where the energies of a charismatic performer could produce visible effects among members of the audience.

Miracle tales of supernatural powers of healing or paranormal abilities attained through practice or from a special master sparked the urban imagination. Qigong healing narratives seemed boundless, full of exuberant, sometimes fantastic tales. Stories of miraculous healing sessions where paralyzed people who had been wheeled or carried in by relatives could suddenly walk by themselves without any aid and accounts of the magical powers of masters who could turn on light bulbs in their bare hands circulated at work units, in hospital lines, or on morning strolls. Mr. Wang, a factory worker in his fifties, related how he, a nonpractitioner, had been convinced that qigong worked:

> I didn't really believe in qigong or know much about it. My mother [in her eighties] had heard about a famous master coming to Beijing and mentioned interest in going to the event. I didn't plan to go, but somehow our relatives managed to get some complimentary tickets through their work unit and gave them to us. I'm the eldest son, so she lives with us now, and if she needs to go out, I have to carry her to my bike cart and pedal her myself. So we went to hear Master Zhang. The stadium was packed with people who had

paid twenty yuan each. When he began to lecture, some people started to rock back and forth. Eventually, my mother, who has severe arthritis but is mentally clear, stood up and began to wave her arms. It's painful for her to stand on her bound feet for long, but that night she stood four hours, the entire time of the lecture. Now I don't have to carry her around anymore. She likes to walk around the neighborhood and go out every day with a cane. It's like watching a young kid.

Whether or not people fully believed in qigong or practiced regularly, the changes they saw in others or felt themselves were convincing enough. Healing narratives were an integral component of the spread of qigong. Such stories, presenting proof of the authenticity and power of a particular form or master, were crucial in winning over skeptics.

Like Mr. Wang's mother, most individuals took up qigong as part of a longer search for healing after life-threatening illness. In a chance meeting over lunch with Dan Dan, a friend's cousin in her thirties, the conversation turned to qigong. Dan Dan did not practice any form of qigong but believed completely in its healing powers. She indicated, "If you want to know why this is so hot, you should talk to my mom. She cured her own cancer, and now people are coming to see her for advice about their illnesses." Several weeks later we met with her mother over a simple lunch of tomato-egg soup, stir-fried eggplant, and *lao bing* (northern Chinese fried dough). A petite woman in her late sixties, Mrs. Huang walked with a lively gait and sat on a small folding stool with her hands resting palms up on her knees while talking.

> I practice walking qigong and do so for about forty minutes a day. I started learning in 1978 to cure myself of cancer. The hospital didn't take in severe cases then, so even after thirty years of service, we [cancer patients] still couldn't find a place to die. There was an article by Huang Song Xiao, who talked about how cancer can be cured with qigong and gave sample medical histories. Once I started, my tumor shrank and then disappeared. In 1982 I toured after my recovery. People who heard about my illness wanted me to write them but it's easier to give demonstrations in person. So since then, I've traveled to Dalian, Shenyang, Qiqihar, Shanghai, Wuxi, even the oilfields in Daqing. I've been invited all over the country, even to hospitals. Most people take on qigong to cure themselves like me.

After describing the normal responses to qigong, such as tears, sweat, mucous, pain, and prickling sensations, she proceeded to give a demonstration of her walking qigong. In a very stylized, slow walk across the tiny apartment, she moved her arms deliberately from side to side showing how to exhale and inhale along the way. She continued, "Your mind and body need to be united to cure yourself. Wherever your thoughts go, qi goes also. In order to undergo self-healing, it's important for the mind and body to work together. One should practice every day from 5 A.M. to 7 A.M. and then at night before sleeping. I practice lying down."

Mrs. Huang's determination to survive her brain tumor led her to try alternatives after she was denied brain surgery. Her success subsequently led many other patients and family members to seek her out. She found a new calling, lecturing on her method of self-healing. Stories such as hers traveled quickly, spread not only by word of mouth but also by state media and semiprivate journals that fanned the flames of popular interest.

QIGONG FEVER IN MASS MEDIA

The conversations in parks and group healing demonstrations, which focused on communal practice and self-healing, were amplified in the wider realm of state publishing and media. *In the Red*, Geremie Barmé's (1999) account of the publication frenzy in China during the late twentieth century, gives a sense of how many journals, books, and publications, both official and unofficial, were consumed there during this period. One central distinction of the post-Mao qigong craze in contrast to earlier millenarian movements was its promulgation among urban-based citizens, especially elites such as intellectuals, scientists, and cadres. Much of this popularity was supported and promoted by passionate reportage in news media, intense debates published in journals, magazines, and even state dailies, and the extensive publication of best-sellers by qigong masters. Any book on qigong was a guaranteed hit.

Lydia Liu's (1995) study on translingual practices calls for careful contextualization of the production of knowledge and for the reinsertion of politics and culture in the analysis of such moments. In China, for instance, newsprint articles tended to disseminate official views or report on public events, while a new genre of semiofficial publications emerged on street stands. The same changes that led to the withdrawal of funding for state enterprises such as factories and hospitals pressured publishing houses to develop marketing strategies to ensure viability. Controls over content and political correctness were relaxed. This was partly due to the general perception at the time that qigong addressed concerns about healing and hence was apolitical. Following popular interest would ensure a return on one's investment.

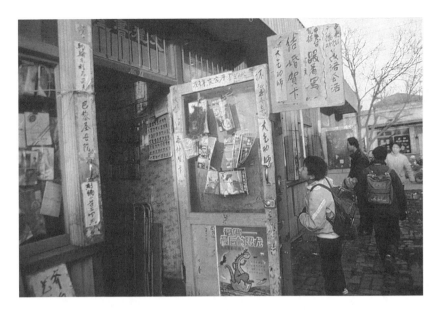

9. Bookstore in 1990 with handwritten display of best-sellers. One of the titles featured is *Da qigongshi* (Great qigong master).

The move to privatization by state publishing houses meant that more best-sellers would be needed to bring in revenue. Publishing houses, once under the rule of propaganda bureaus, could publish best-sellers rather than politically correct or "red" texts, and this paved the way for the publication of popular texts on health and medicine. Small book stalls and magazine stands stocked with glossy beauty magazines and new journals such as *Xiandai Qigong* (Contemporary qigong) and *Qigong Shijie* (Qigong world) proliferated (see figs. 9 and 10). State newspapers like *Renmin Ribao* (People's daily) and local dailies such as *Beijing Wanbao* (Beijing evening daily) also reported on qigong. Most daily newspapers in China comprise four to ten pages at most, so such texts tended to offer condensed accounts focusing on qigong as martial art, meditation, and breathing exercise. Still, some articles on the specific styles associated with certain masters publicized more charismatic forms of the practice.

As private and state publishers began to bring out more books about qigong, martial art novels, and spiritual texts, and as mass media accounts of the boom in qigong practice spread across the country, the interest in qigong eventually became a national obsession. Images of powerful masters and the miracles of qigong healing abounded both in popular films and novels. Inside

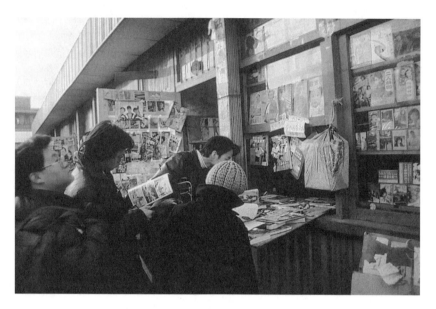

10. More book stalls, these selling popular magazines

the state-owned bookstore on Wangfujing Street in Beijing during the 1990s, readers could find a variety of books about qigong. Chinese texts presented instructional, autobiographical, historical, fictional, and scientific writing. A few state publishing houses produced books with simple instructions and diagrams of specific postures and movements. Books on qigong generally cost about 10 to 25 yuan (around $3 U.S. in 1990, or about a day's wage for the average factory worker).[7]

Autobiographical texts tended to begin with up to a dozen photos of the qigong master in tranquil poses or together with famous movie stars or state leaders. The inclusion of such celebrities conferred status and legitimacy on the master. Also vital to the autobiographical genre was the origin narrative, which revealed the life history of the master and, more important, how he or she came to recognize and cultivate special qigong powers. Remaining chapters included case histories of patients cured by the master's healing abilities. Biographies of three major qigong masters who were known throughout China sold out immediately, and hard-to-find dog-eared copies were passed from friend to friend. Historical texts about qigong by Chinese scholars tended to emphasize the more-than-five-thousand-year history of qi cultivation. Though "qigong" is by all accounts a neologism that only became popular in the mid-twentieth century, many historical accounts merged qi cultivation exercises of past spiritual and Daoist ritual practices with contemporary qigong. Such linkages with the past were also made in the popular realm.

Perhaps even more popular than the autobiographies of qigong masters are the martial art novellas and comic books (*wuxia xiaosuo*) on which many a martial art film has been based. Ke Yunlu, nom de plume of a popular writing team, wrote the runaway best-seller of 1989, *Da Qigong Shi* (Great qigong master), enthralling readers with tales of a qigong master's adventures in the city as he searched for truth and universal forces. The satirical fictional account explicated the roots of qigong in philosophy and Daoism. Following the literary conventions of a martial arts novel, the story traces a typical master's rise to power as he encounters people as diverse as students, workers, peasants, middle-level bureaucrats, and cadres. The social worlds of qigong that the author described paralleled the immense following that feverishly attended mass qigong sessions and sought out masters in the parks. Sold out immediately, copies of *Da Qigong Shi* passed along networks of friends, coworkers, and neighbors. Each time I inquired about the book, friends and colleagues had just lent their own copies to someone else. Readers from all walks of life found the satirical sketches to be a daring social commentary not just about practitioners but also about the upper echelons of leadership. But state officials found the novel painted too sardonic a picture of contemporary life, and a year after its publication book stalls were raided and larger bookstores were asked to remove the book from the shelves.

QIGONG IN THE SCIENTIFIC COMMUNITY

Qigong began to be actively debated within the scientific community during the 1980s, when scientists, especially physicists, sought to legitimate the phenomenon of qi. While popular publications focused on practice or gave life histories of particular masters, the discussions of qigong among scientists addressed questions of how to measure the force field of qi energy. Qi as a material phenomenon had to be quantified. This interest paralleled attention to the phenomenon of *teyigongneng*, or special psychic abilities. Many scholars and bureaucrats mentioned how the doors of scientific research opened when Qian Xuesen, the prominent founder of China's space research termed the father of the Chinese missile, declared in the 1980s that teyigongneng merited serious study. In his account of this movement, Paul Dong, a

U.S.–based qigong master, described how young children in China were test-ed for their abilities to "hear" characters being written and to perform psy-chokinesis (the power to move objects with the minds); there were reports of pills disappearing from bottles only to materialize outside their containers (Dong and Raffill 1997). Scientific experiments with qigong masters also com-menced during this period, as many researchers and practitioners believed that special abilities could be enhanced with qigong. Over a dozen scientific jour-nals and publications, among them, *Zhiran Zazhi* (Nature magazine) and *Dongfang Qigong* (Eastern qigong), began to discuss human potential and somatic science. What was at stake was Chinese scientists' affirmation of tra-ditional forms of knowledge and phenomena. Whereas popular journals fol-lowed public interest, the scientific community was grappling with how to describe qi phenomena. The much-publicized scientific debates in newspapers and journals had wide impact. Their appearance in state media suggested the official sanction of the state.[8] Ultimately, qigong research led to new scientific discourses that would eventually be used to regulate masters who were believed to promote unscientific forms of qigong, but, for the moment, science seemed to be as taken with the practice as the public at large.

Fevers reveal an important relation between social interest and state desires. Sometimes, as in the early development of qigong, these coincide such that fevers flourish as state-sanctioned projects. Qigong fever, in particular, offered different spaces in which it was possible to experience alternate realities apart from the state.

In what follows, I examine the role that qigong masters played in the emer-gence of new subjectivities.

CHAPTER THREE

RIDING THE TIGER

A PRACTITIONER'S ABILITIES were intricately linked to those of his or her teacher. Masters were not only adept in healing and the movement of qi; they were also viewed as the ultimate embodiment of power. This chapter examines the naturalized powers of these individuals, asking how they became established authorities. A 1990 Chinese political cartoon shows a generic, aged state bureaucrat unwittingly holding the tail of a tiger that is turning to pounce back on him. In contrast, qigong masters were said to embody the ultimate ability to "ride the tiger," that is, to master difficult situations rather than being overwhelmed by them. The norms of being in control and capable of maintaining rightful power were especially questioned in the post-1989 Tiananmen period. Masters were believed to be able to immerse themselves in chaos and emerge with true power in health and wealth. By being in control of both material wealth and symbolic capital, they were capable of upstaging state leaders. Not only could they harness tremendous powers and thus garner thousands of followers, even numbering state officials among them, they were widely viewed as having the ultimate powers that qi energy could bring: longevity, prosperity, and superhuman abilities. In sum, these people accumulated power in a period when capital, both material and symbolic, became increasingly more crucial to one's status and the social economy. During public performances, masters were the center of attention, whether they lectured on the healing powers of qi or energetically demonstrated such abilities. In parks, masters were equally charismatic as they healed patients surrounded by intimate groups of supplicants. In this chapter, I trace the careers of three such individuals. These masters went beyond the ordinary circuits of simply teaching qigong. They were able to parlay their social networks into extensive entrepreneurial enterprises in the new economy while promoting a traditional form of healing.

The category of tradition is not a unified or stable category, as other anthropologists of China have shown. Whether in the hinterlands or in urban centers, different cultural agents and producers actively engage in appropriating meanings of tradition and authenticity that are distinct from state discourses of modernity. Ralph Litzinger notes in his study of the Yao ethnic minority and their local ethnological practices that " 'traditional culture,' or *chuantong wenhua*, became an object to be managed as intellectuals, scholars, and party cadres worked to define the correct relationship between 'traditional culture' and socialist modernity" (2000, 240). Similarly, in her study of ethnic minority cultural politics, Louisa Schein comments that, "in fact, tradition was being vigorously recuperated by Miao cultural practitioners" (2000, 284). In the urban context, qigong masters came to represent traditional or indigenous knowledge of healing. The power to heal drew on a long-standing history and social imagination about adepts. The influence of masters on those in power reached far back to imperial courts, where emperors interested in longevity had their own Daoist *fangshi* (recipe masters) as alchemy consultants (Harper 1998).

Healing in the immediate post-Mao period, before the formation of a massive market economy in the 1990s, emerged simultaneously as a private practice of cultivation for individuals and a public performance for masters. In contrast to previous decades, where socialized medicine attended to the masses, in the 1980s qigong emerged in response to desires for individualized forms of healing in the face of the changing health care system. It promised release and hope: elderly people could attend to their rheumatism or arthritis, long-term sufferers of neurasthenia or chronic pain could seek relief, and even parents of children with congenital disorders could seek help when no other options could be found in either traditional Chinese medicine or biomedicine. Whether in parks or in stadiums, qigong made it possible to cry openly or express fervent belief in something outside state ideology. As some forms of qigong began to overlap with Daoist, Buddhist, and other spiritual practices, references to qigong as a religion or new age spiritualism emerged.

Popular narratives about qigong emphasized the fantastic and superhuman powers of qigong and its masters. In the initial period of accommodation (1983–1990), official state discourse seemed to mirror the public view that qigong was miraculous and even took steps to co-opt it as a state treasure. Each week, broadcasts on radio and television in addition to print media ranging from state news organs to magazines carried stories of people cured of terminal diseases or of masters demonstrating their special skills. Many individuals stepped forward to show off their skills in parks or, if they had greater capabilities, to perform publicly in larger arenas. Rumors about qigong powers circulated quickly, not only via media channels but also by word of mouth on buses, trains, and planes across the country. Concerns about superstitious practices were less important during this period, when a resurgence of traditional rituals and practices occurred throughout rural and urban areas. Masters occupied the public, semiofficial space of social imagination and came to embody an ultimate form of personal power.

By the late 1980s, the stage was set for several charismatic qigong masters, who captured the popular imagination with their powers to heal and bring thousands in an audience to states of trance and ecstatic movement. Charmed followers reported miraculous transformations from illness to well-being and newfound meaning in daily practice. Factory workers and cadres alike paid 35 to 40 yuan (the equivalent of a week's wages) to attend mass sessions conducted by famous masters in hopes of receiving the master's external (*wai*) qi. Meanwhile, traveling shows of less well known qigong magicians (*moshu*) adept at feats of external qi energy held performances on streets or in work units that included walking on glass and later swallowing the shards, feeling no pain from fire or great blows to the body, or demonstrating special abilities such as hearing written characters. Yet, as public spaces became disengaged from official state discourses, many qigong practitioners still felt the need to legitimate their practices through official recognition, for example, by registering for licenses to practice with the state qigong administration bureau.

QIGONG AND THE PARANORMAL

Tales of supernatural entities and powers have infused popular literary themes and vernacular culture in China for centuries. Despite various campaigns to eradicate interest or belief in the occult during both the Republican era (1930s) and the Cultural Revolution (1965–75), the fascination with paranormal phenomena has continued in post-Mao China. Before discussing how qigong masters become charismatic leaders, it is crucial to differentiate the closely related phenomena of psychic or paranormal abilities referred to as teyigongneng from qigong.

Mr. Bao was a reputed master of paranormal abilities and even considered to be a state treasure. He did not practice qigong, and neither was he considered to be a qigong master. His abilities to make things disappear or materialize were considered to be natural talents (*tiancai*). A common tale that spread around Beijing was that he could easily make a coin disappear from a subject's hand and make it reappear in the person's belly. Though many qigong masters arguably have such abilities, and their demonstration in public performances contributed to the popular conception of them as superhuman. Phantasmagoric stories of how a particular master could walk or see right through walls or make pills pop out of unopened bottles spread like wildfire across China. The range of extraordinary abilities included such extrasensory abilities as hearing sounds from far away, smelling fragrances from a different, closed room, enhancing the taste of foods or smells of objects, and identifying written characters without seeing the words. In *China's Super Psychics*, Paul Dong (and Raffill 1997), a qigong master who has lived in the United States for several decades, contends that children are the most likely to experience paranormal or psychic abilities as innate qualities. The belief in such powers easily extended beyond small circles of practitioners, circulating widely in both popular and official circuits.

Some scientists considered qigong to be a natural phenomena in the same category as teyigongneng. Special research institutes emerged in the 1980s devoted to conducting experiments on individuals with special talents such as the ability to move objects with qi, to charge the human body and other objects with electricity, to "read" Chinese characters with the ears, or to heal individuals. Another camp of scientists went even further, taking the extreme position that qigong was a precious Chinese tradition that needed to be protected as a state secret. One master reputed to have supernatural powers was sequestered under tight security so that his abilities could be further researched. Popular rumors circulated of how the master terrorized his bodyguards with threats of qi-induced bodily harm.

Nearly all martial art novels and films feature figures who can see or even walk through walls, transport objects with mind power, and enter other spiritual worlds or dimensions. The scientific community throughout the provinces pursued studies of such phenomenon. In the late 1970s and throughout the 1980s many notable scientists started such investigations, holding conferences on psychic abilities and debating the scientific qualities of paranormal power. Similar investigations took place in the Soviet Union during the height of the cold war. My intention here is to distinguish the general debates about psychic power from the parallel discussions about qigong masters. Though the intertwining phenomena of psychics and powerful masters emerged simultaneously in the post-Mao context, the social life and career trajectories of masters were different. The powers of the majority of children with psychic abilities are reported to fade in adulthood. In contrast, masters with no innate capabilities have fostered or cultivated their abilities by learning qigong later in life. More-over, if they chose to pursue healing as a career, they continued to attain pow-ers beyond psychic powers. In sum, rather than becoming subjects to observe and record, such masters transcended the ordinary world.

As a cultural phenomenon studied by anthropologists at the turn of the cen-tury, magic was considered to be characteristic of primitive societies where sci-ence had not yet replaced traditional structures of knowledge and power. A similar view of magic was adopted in the People's Republic during the early Maoist years, when magic was associated with superstition (*mixin*) and back-wardness (*luohou*). Campaigns against mixin during the Cultural Revolution targeted traditional and spiritual practices that were believed to hold the na-tion back from achieving modernization. These practices included qigong, which had a brief moment during the 1950s, when Liu Guizheng, an official representative, toured the country to explain to party cadres and urbanites the powers of healing with qi. According to informants who practiced before the post-Mao economic reforms, the political atmosphere of the 1960s and 1970s made qigong (and any personal pursuits) nearly impossible for fear that they would be mistaken for spiritual practices and lack of political fervor. The re-framing of qigong as a healing art and science rather than an offshoot of the more magical category of teyigongneng during the economic reforms made it possible for people to participate.

MASTERING THE MEDIA

By the early 1990s qigong had grown into a widespread social phenomenon with a broad base of followers and masters both in and outside China. The proliferation of practitioners was especially visible after the Tianan-men demonstrations and before state economic policies began to be renewed. Enterprising masters became charismatic cultural producers of healing and even modern-day mystics or shamans traveling a transnational circuit. Individuals who claimed to be masters of healing opened clinics or charged dearly for pri-vate sessions. Masters were the embodiment of entrepreneurial spirit as they mobilized local forms of networks (*guanxi*) as well as new technologies (the Internet) to expand their enterprises. The appeal of these masters depended less on their personalities than on the actual effects they had on people. Such charisma could not only be found on the stages from which masters presented lectures to large audiences but also amplified in the media, and effectively nav-igating and even managing local media became a means for masters to legitimize themselves. In previous decades, all media were considered to be owned by the state and promoted state rhetoric; the winds of political change could be noted simply by reading the editorials of key publications such as *Renmin Ribao* (People's daily). During the Tiananmen demonstrations, articulations of a fragmented, even dissenting press revealed possibilities for a mass media based on popular interests. In the Deng reforms, official media still retained their role as the voice of state leaders; however, new publications aimed at a popular readership for profit turned toward more lucrative figures such as masters. In addition to specialized magazines and journals such as *Qigong Science*, mainstream newspapers began to include daily articles on masters.

The wide appeal of qigong encouraged coverage in a diverse array of print and television sources, not all of them expressing state-sanctioned views, though even central state media devoted a fair amount of attention to this latest craze. Many journalists underwent qigong healing or attended mass demonstrations.[2] Chinese television, like its print counterparts, was restricted to specific news. Qigong, however, viewed by state officials as a traditional healing art, was considered to be acceptable news. The visual impact of watching masters flick on unattached light bulbs or using the power of qi to command physically impaired individuals to walk was extraordinary. Broadcasting these miracles tended to give them the stamp of authenticity, playing on notions that seeing is believing. One master in his late sixties enjoyed a fifteen-minute segment demonstrating qigong practice on state television. Such coverage ensured an even greater audience. Outside official networks, other visual media also began to circulate, promoting masters' powers and social capital. Videos produced privately by masters and sold at lectures or independently produced could be obtained commercially, primarily reaching urbanites with disposable income. Masters who toured the country giving lectures sold audio- and videotapes to generate additional profits. These videos reached an audience composed primarily of urbanites with disposable income. Videos, like books and audiotapes, aided in promoting a master's powers and social capital.

Though most privately produced videos unabashedly extolled the virtues of qigong healing and the abilities of masters, one noteworthy exception countered these claims. Mr. Ma, a former master, came to disbelieve in some masters' claims to cure anything. A journalist trained in economics, he took up martial arts and external qigong as a side interest. Eventually, Ma began to publish articles in state newspapers denouncing false practices. He then decided to make a video that would reveal some of the secrets of qigong. The filming took place at a local high school in front of an audience of teachers. Ma disguised himself as a peasant master who could accomplish a variety of fantastic deeds: swallowing glass, breaking bricks with his body, breathing fire, holding back motorcycles or vans with his teeth, emitting qi to a television, and much more. Later, he returned to the camera wearing a Western suit and tie to discuss how each feat was actually accomplished. The effect of his transformation from an illiterate peasant to an articulate urbanite espousing scientific rationality was so stunning that the Chinese government eventually appropriated the video, producing and distributing it as an official debunking tool. It was shown on Chinese Central Television, and videos were sold at state-run bookstores for 100 yuan (about a month's salary). Official embrace of the video was accompanied by attacks from other masters for its demystification of qigong healing: ultimately, Ma and his family faced death threats. Still, his exposé of masters who were powerful social brokers led to a subsequent career as a cult buster.

In response to the proliferation of charismatic masters who operated without responsibility to any official unit, state regulation was initiated. Citing qigong deviation and "false," unscientific practices as reasons for state intervention, steps were undertaken to license masters and prevent popular mass sessions. But even though practitioners and the social context of qigong came under scrutiny by state regulatory bureaus, individuals and state officials alike continued to practice the breathing and healing exercises, sometimes deliberately in defiance of growing rules or simply with the rationale that leisure hours devoted to self-healing were apolitical.

LEAVING THE MOUNTAIN: WAYS TO BECOME A MASTER

In the course of my interviews with qigong practitioners and patients, many referred to their masters in reverent tones. After regaling me with their own stories of being healed, followers would continue with the saga of how their masters emerged from the mountains (*chushanle*) or became semipublic figures. "Chushanle" refers to Buddhist and Daoist traditions of retreating to mountainous monasteries or the great wilderness for cultivation and spiritual development. Retreat meant leaving a world of immoral conflict and strife to seek restoration of the mind and body. Return to the everyday world meant that a person had a moral obligation or purpose to fulfill. Qigong masters and practitioners frequently termed leaving the mountain the key moment in their development as healers, when they assumed the mantles of responsibility passed on to them by their teachers or spiritual guides. The timing of their emergence is linked to vast economic and social changes.

Operating within a post-Mao economy led to the emergence of different types of masters. Whereas previously most were martial artists or traditional

medical healers, in the 1990s the entrepreneurial master who healed with qi became prominent. In the numerous interviews I had with masters and teachers
of varied forms, I often asked how they became masters. From what I observed
in public parks, this category seemed quite flexible, as though anyone could
claim to be a master (*shi*). Not all masters had the same capabilities, however,
and the number of followers varied accordingly. Especially because practitioners could self-heal, the possession of "true" qigong capabilities (*gongneng*) to exert qi and heal others was frequently invoked as a primary characteristic of a
master. It was not unusual in the early 1990s to see individuals lined up each
morning to seek diagnosis and prompt healing with qi by a master reputed to
have special powers.

The path to becoming a master has several stages. Just as they follow numerous forms, the masters of each type also vary greatly in age and abilities.
One first becomes a practitioner and chooses whether to remain secluded in
one's practice or train for living in the mundane world. Although both males
and females can practice, males are more likely to train as masters because of
the patrilineal nature of knowledge transfer. If a practitioner is lucky, a master
of a particular tradition recognizes in him or her abilities worthy of further
training. After many years of training as a disciple, individuals branch out by
doing good deeds with their powers. This is often referred to as "leaving the
mountain" of seclusion and entering the everyday world. It is crucial at this
time to prove that one can heal others with the power of qi from one's body.

The majority of masters and healers that I interviewed (90 percent) mentioned self-healing as their primary motivation for beginning to practice. Their
stories of overcoming severe or chronic illnesses mirrored the stories of ordinary practitioners told in chapter 2. Master Song, in his youthful seventies, began practicing for better energy and to keep his qi "open" to cure his neurasthenia in the 1960s. Originally a cadre, he retired after becoming a healer.
Speaking from his modest courtyard home of forty-five years where he and his
wife practiced daily, he outlined three types of qi: *yunqi*, which refers to one's
fortune; *lianqi*, indicating Buddhist and Daoist forms that require practice;
and *yangqi*, which nurtures growth and development. In summarizing these
distinct forms, he restated the importance of breath, "No matter what type of
qigong, we can't be separated from breath [*huxi*]." Though he was much
younger, in his midthirties, Master Chen suffered from ulcers and had been
hospitalized eight times for this painful condition. In 1983 he began to study
hexiangzhuang gong, which helped him overcome his illness and continue in his
day job as a factory worker. Master Dong, in his sixties, suffered from metasta-
tic cancer and had surgery five times to remove tumors. He also began practice
in 1983, at the Shanghai athletic qigong course. In the mornings he practiced

donggong (moving qigong) to cure his illness, while in the evenings he engaged in *jingong* (meditation qigong) to relax his mind and body. After suffering from severe disease, Master Dong felt much more sensitive to the illness of others. "I am very perceptive and can diagnose patients from a distance. For instance, I can find cancer or check the liver. My diagnostic technique is different from the hospital, but I'm usually correct." Healing narratives from masters indicated a growing recognition of special abilities to heal others.

During the 1990s it became easier to open qigong schools without coming from a traditional line of masters and to train even those students who lacked such lineage themselves. Even so, being a descendant of a practice lineage continued to be a way to become a master. As with other forms of martial arts and Daoist or Buddhist practices, the world of qigong had multiple forms or styles of practice with different masters embodying particular schools or lineages of training. Just as they follow numerous forms, so the masters of each type vary greatly in age and abilities. A common term used to refer to the descendants of a particular master was "*tudi*," indicating a special disciple or apprentice who would eventually inherit the master's special knowledge and even his followers in the event of his passing. Most disciples tended to be male, in keeping with the traditional forms of patrilineal descent, although sometimes fathers wished to pass on their skills to their daughters as well. Regardless, as one practitioner cautioned me, "even if a master has several tudi, the master may never tell which one who will be the ultimate inheritor of his special skills until the very end. Or they may never find out and will have to contest each other until the most powerful disciple wins out." This strategy ensured that a master would remain in power until his time was up. This structure of relations between disciples and master also meant that, even within the same generation, each student could have quite different levels of skill and knowledge.

Master Dong, who had survived cancer, described how he established himself:

> I was in the first qigong class at the Shanghai Municipal Sports Commission. It was a teacher's training course, and we were told to go forth and teach others. Students come by after seeing advertisements in the papers or by introduction. The average is about forty-four persons. I've already taught over seven thousand students. At first, tuition was three yuan, then six yuan, and now it's thirty yuan per month. We started out with a three-month course, but now we have a two-month course for advanced students. All the instructors are licensed from the 1983 course, but we have to go to Beijing to recertify ourselves every few years. The exam has a written and an oral component, but it's based on personal experience as well.

The secularized model of learning made it possible for masters to teach far more students in the emergent category of masters as instructors as opposed to masters as healers.

In addition to the two more common pathways to power mentioned above, another recent pathway to masterhood involved establishing a network of clients that subscribed to the healing powers of the master. The more powerful and well connected the clients, the more prestige the master accumulated. Hence status was a reflection more of secular power than of the relative powers of a master. Nevertheless, this strategy became a prominent path to power. In many masters' autobiographies and popular qigong manuals, photographs of the master taken with state leaders, intellectuals, or even movie stars are prominently displayed in the first pages. Such displays signified that the masters had the tacit if not official recognition of state representatives.

Qigong practitioners come from all backgrounds, and males and females are equally represented. At the level of qigong master, however, there are significantly fewer women. Though I have met many of these, I contend that qigong masters have come to represent a naturalized category of masculinity and that forms of qigong practice are gendered in the social context. How did qigong become affiliated with masculinity? I propose that while popular images of masculinity seem to be based on social abilities and external physical features, notions of the properties of qi attributable to physiology that circulate in discourses of qigong further underscore Chinese notions of masculinity. Moreover, in the public display of qigong there is a heightened sense of hypermasculinity, with practitioners appearing to have superhuman powers of invulnerability and longevity. In my research, I found that the gendered hierarchy of healing ability—that is, the presence of more male qigong masters—was due to both physiological explanations and social discourses. Gender and qi can be linked in traditional Chinese medicine, but I argue that it is not only the corporeal discourses of qi that account for the overwhelming number of male masters but also the social context and performances of qigong that specifically associate qi with male essence. In the 1990s particular individuals emerged as masters who embodied naturalized categories of qigong masculinity. It is crucial to acknowledge the social relations of power in which the expression of qigong healing and power articulated a political cosmology of qi in addition to the natural cosmology.

Despite the multitude of styles and genealogies of practice, qigong can be distinguished into two types, external and internal, both with gender characteristics. The external form, *ying gong* (sometimes referred to as hard qigong), tends to emphasize hard qi and hard bodies that can withstand much force and perform superhuman acts. This martial form tends to be practiced not so much in public parks as on streets, in acrobatic troupes, or even in military compounds. One well-known master told me he would often be invited to give special qigong training sessions for the public security forces and People's Liberation Army troops. The masters and practitioners of this form are primarily men, and masculine displays of power are a factor in the performance of qigong. In contrast, the internal and meditative form, *neigong*, tends to attract female practitioners. It is not unusual to find practitioners of both genders and all backgrounds practicing this form in parks, however: internal forms of cultivation and qigong also greatly appeal to male practitioners, as they promote the circulation and transformation of qi and blood, crucial steps toward enhancing male potency and preventing pathologies such as seminal emission or sexual impotence. Despite the existence of an extensive range of aphrodisiacs and male potency-enhancing remedies, qigong practice was cheaper and more effective in the long term. Both forms of qigong, then, carry appeal for men, the one responding to the desire for an impenetrable hard body and the other offering self-generating potency.

In her analysis of the quest for masculinity in post-Mao literature, Xueping Zhong (2000) notes that certain elements of masculinity were being reworked and debated during the late 1980s and 1990s. Specific players, whom she refers to as "male intellectual/critics," have been key agents in the formation of Chinese modernity and discourses of masculinity. The *xungen* (search for roots) literary movement was a "conflation of search for roots and male self" (154). The literary obsession with potency was also reflected in the formation of *nanke*, the specialization of male pathology (Farquhar 1999). Anagnost describes the xungen movement as a "nostalgic retrieval of a great Chinese civilization of the past" (1997, 154). The specter of impotence emerged simultaneously with the transformation of medicine and gender under market reform. Nanke reflected an obsession with the symptoms of powerlessness while also fostering new forms of consumption. Concerns about masculinity in the new economy further fueled interest in qigong promoted by masters adept in superhuman abilities.

Traditionally, there are two levels of masters. The term *shi*, used in spiritual and martial arts circles, forms part of the terms for both teacher (*laoshi*) and master (*shifu*). An emergent category of *dashi* (great master) was used to indicate those who rose beyond teaching and healing to accumulate vast material resources and social capital. Situating oneself within a lineage of qigong knowledge and practice was a crucial marker of authenticity and rightful power. One could bypass this process by demonstrating special abilities and establishing oneself through a base of clientele. The more famous the client, the more prestige this reflected back on the master. In addition, fostering disciples, key individuals who helped to organize and disseminate one's teaching and reputation, was crucial. In the rapid embrace of consumer culture and the market economy, promotion of a master often entailed frequent tours throughout the country. In addition to admission fees, books, photographs, audiotapes, videos, and other qigong practice aids were crucial materials both to gain publicity and to generate income. An overseas connection was crucial to making the big time. Whether as an official delegate to demonstrate qigong as part of a Chinese entourage or via private sponsors, going abroad offered significant social and material consequences. The circulation of masters in a global context amplified an already significant alternative economy of bodies and desires that were emerging in post-Mao China.

MASTERS OF THE UNIVERSE

In 1991 three major figures captured the public imagination, discussed in both official state discourse and the popular realm. Their different fates illustrate the ambivalent relations the Chinese government had with qigong masters and the way in which their allegiances transformed their careers. One emigrated to the United States, another was sent to prison, and the third went into exile in Sichuan Province.

The first, Dr. Zheng, a traditional medical doctor and the descendant of a well-known master, received wide acclaim during the 1980s and was generally accepted by the intellectual and bureaucratic elite since he spoke as a licensed medical healer. Told by his master to spread the word and continue his lineage, Dr. Zheng began in 1983 to lecture on qigong. Word of his stamina and abilities spread rapidly, not least because his marathon lectures often lasted five to six hours without pause, even for a sip of water. Magazines such as *Huacheng* declared him to be "China's superman" (cited in Zhu 1990, 10). In his initial ascent, he published numerous books and participated in the first scientific experiments on qi at Qinghua University, often referred to as the MIT of China. Lending credence to his form were his insistence on scientific proof and his alliances with rational bureaucrats. His followers kept in touch via an email list server and met regularly in meetings across the United States and Canada. In the late eighties, he managed to get a visa to the United States and has since acquired new audiences and followers for his practice.

The fate of the second master, who became infamous in post-Mao China, is particularly instructive. Ms. Xu was a woman master in her late thirties who quickly amassed an overwhelming popular base and impressive material wealth. An outsider in Beijing, she had few connections to upper echelons of the state bureaucracy. Rather than being a personal healer ministering to the chronic ailments of state officials, she focused her attention on an immense base of everyday citizens (*laobaixing*), who attended her lectures religiously, eagerly paying 35 yuan for each ticket (equivalent to one week's salary for an urban worker in 1990). Youthful and vivacious, a former actress with the Qinghai Performance Troupe, she claimed to have been bestowed with special powers to heal others and the ability to speak in tongues, or "universal language" (*yuzhouyu*). Her vision of the universe as a new creation of humanity and other aspects of her spiritual journey and enlightenment were documented in her autobiographical novel *Da Ziran De Hunpo* (The soul of the natural world, 1989). She accumulated a large following, ranging from cadres and professionals to workers and chronically ill of both genders and all ages. In the former Temple of Heaven, followers of her style would move in qigong-induced trances around a big tree that was said to be infused with her qi. At the height of her popularity, several hundred people would go to this tree to practice collectively and speak in tongues.

In spite of the ban on large public gatherings during martial law following the Tiananmen demonstrations, this master managed to hold a series of qigong sessions in March 1990 using the upcoming Asian Games as justification for a fundraiser that generated over a million yuan. Over several nights, Ms. Xu lectured to several thousand participants eager to hear her speak and receive energy (*shou gong*). Shortly after her performance, many individuals claimed to be able to speak in tongues and have visions of ancestral spirits or the master herself. Outpatient clinics at mental wards were suddenly deluged with concerned relatives who brought in patients suffering from hallucinations and disruptive behavior associated with attending Xu's session. In the weeks following this performance, editorials in *Renmin Ribao* (People's daily) and *Jiankang Ribao* (Health daily) began to question Master Xu's motives and responsibility in bringing such large numbers of people to uncontrollable emotional outbursts and mass hysteria.[3] Accusations of witchcraft and superstition began to emerge. Xu was called *wupo* (witch) and *pianzi* (swindler) and accused of dabbling in *mixin* and *shenmi* (mysticism) with her forms of *xie* (evil) qi. It was clear that, for the authorities, her form of qigong, with its apocalyptic statements about the existing regime, had too much in common with evangelical faith-healing meetings and heterodox cult groups.

When several patients who had sought her healing powers died shortly afterward, Beijing municipal authorities called for her arrest and charged her with healing without a license. In the summer of 1990, Ms. Xu was convicted of these charges. Her imprisonment was widely publicized, leaving in its wake a broad wave of concern among practitioners and other masters. Negative news coverage of Xu was limited to official media such as the *Renmin Ribao*), *Jiankang Ribao*, and *Falu Shenhuo Zhazi* (Law and life). Such media took the now-official stance toward the regulation of qigong. Not all journalists took the hard line immediately. For some who practiced qigong themselves, their publications on the topic revealed an ambivalent approach to the neo-Confucian overtures of the state. Physicians and public health authorities also demanded the regulation of qigong to diminish the involvement of charlatans. Soon it became clear that to continue to practice as either master or student, one would have to register and pay regular dues to an officially sanctioned school.

In the months following Xu's arrest, many masters either positioned themselves within official boundaries or went underground. At the big tree to which Master Xu attributed special powers, only a handful of the most devoted practitioners continued to meet in the later part of 1991. Throughout parks one could see red and yellow banners indicating official forms of qigong practice (*zheng qigong*). While the Chinese socialist state viewed the matter as an issue of public health and mass hysteria, the response from the individual practitioner was outrage and indignation. "How dare they lock her up!" a woman cadre in her late fifties responded when I asked her about her practice. She continued, "The reason they locked her up was that she was a woman, and she did not have powerful enough clients to back her up when she started to make a lot of money." Another follower who worked in a mental hospital burst into tears when I inquired about her master. "She did no wrong. Have you heard anything about her?" These deep feelings of concern and sorrow were matched by the opposite reactions of bureaucrats and physicians, who shouted, Xu "is nothing but a modern-day witch."

As an observer in the mental wards, I witnessed concerned family members and physicians who were suddenly confronted with new diagnoses of qigong deviation, the culture-bound syndrome of qigong-induced psychosis. Yet in the parks, among qigong circles, the emerging conclusion was that Xu was being used as a convenient scapegoat by state officials attempting to reassert authority in an arena that was becoming dominated by unlicensed healers. It is important to note the gendered nature of the state-level accusation. During the national campaign denouncing the popular legitimacy of this female master, other masters who operated with a equally large followings managed to escape the label of "modern-day witch" as well as imprisonment. As a female master who managed to attract a popular following, Xu threatened officials, who found her claims unorthodox and unsettling in the political cosmology that had developed over qi and qigong healing. Following her imprisonment, more orthodox and uniform notions of "real" (*zheng*) qigong began to be constructed. The magic of healing from qigong was bound to the claims of the state, which quickly set about distinguishing what it termed orthodox qigong from "false" practices. The example of Ms. Xu was an attempt to rein in masters who seemed to run with the tigers, illustrating how administrators construct notions of unrightful power or the pollution of the powers of qi to serve their own ends.

As Ms. Xu's case was exhibited publicly like "a chicken killed to show the monkeys" (*saji geihoukan*), as one master in the parks neatly put it, the public security bureau was conducting another, more private search to find Mr. Yang, a master in his thirties who was accused of several violent crimes against his followers. He had amassed an immense cult following by setting up a research and healing institute near the Beijing University of Iron and Steel Technology. Unlike his female counterpart, who did not have extensive networks in Beijing, Yang built his empire like a modern-day corporation, complete with his own logo, an autobiographical novel about his spiritual transformation, a monthly newsletter, and a fax number for further contact. His book, which featured the standard array of legitimating photographs of himself with famous personalities and state officials, became a best-seller. With extensive contacts not only in Beijing but in regions far away from the center of bureaucracy, he eventually transferred his base to Sichuan Province, an area where outlaws and dissidents have historically sought refuge. From this base, he allegedly published a series of subversive cartoons lampooning the state officials that called for his arrest (I discuss these in the chapter 6). The public security bureau began an exhaustive search for him, hoping to bring him in for questioning. Eventually, he resurfaced in Guam, where Chinese authorities sought extradition for his criminal activities.

Social and phenomenological discourses about qigong anchor a political cosmology of power in contemporary China. Specific masters have reconfigured meanings of masculinity to include the performativity of both bodily and political prowess. Though certain female masters have challenged the continuities between official and popular meanings of qi, residual images of hypermasculinity remain associated with the practice of qigong and with the intervention of official media and state representatives. Despite their claims of having extraordinary powers, masters still had to establish their authenticity with the bureaucrats intent on regulating their actions in addition to their followers and peers. The campaign to restore social order and the containment of unlicensed but popular masters appeared to be successful. By the summer of 1991 there were no longer vast numbers of qigong practitioners in the parks. Only small groups of elderly people would gather to practice standardized forms more similar to taiji than the ecstatic forms of spontaneous movement that had characterized qigong not long before. The majority of severely ill patients sought healing in official clinics, and large gatherings of any kind had been banned.

Placing masters into binary categories of real or false had profound impact on the feverish interest in qigong. Ultimately, government policy shifted from an initial period of accommodation and state-sanctioned support to a more regulatory stance that involved the medicalization of key behaviors. The next chapter contextualizes the response of the biomedical community to these new disorders.

CHAPTER FOUR

QIGONG DEVIATION OR PSYCHOSIS

SHORTLY AFTER the meteoric rise of qigong practice, individuals began to trickle into traditional medical clinics and biomedical hospitals reporting unusual sensations. Ironically, during the height of the fever some individuals practicing qigong began to experience worrisome bouts of vertigo, uncontrollable qi energy, or disturbing visions. As the popularity of qigong spread in urban centers and rural townships through the media and traveling masters, a related phenomenon began to take place in the psychiatric clinics. Concerned family members or work unit officials began to bring in individuals who complained of misplaced qi energy in their bodies, accompanied by uncontrollable sensations such as extreme heat, hyperactivity, insomnia, hallucinations, or, in some cases, possession. This was usually the last stop on the path of treatment. Most troubled individuals would initially seek help from a master, usually the one with whom they had studied. A master might instruct the practitioner on appropriate techniques to deal with the problem, use his or her own powers of qi to harmonize the disruptive elements within the client (*tiao bing*), or advise the student to discontinue practice altogether. If the symptoms persisted or if family members believed their relatives to be in distress, the next step often involved seeking the help of traditional Chinese medical doctors who specialized in medical qigong. The College of Traditional Chinese Medicine in Beijing and most hospitals offered clinics with this specialty. According to Elizabeth Hsu (1999), qigong was retained under the rubric of traditional Chinese medicine rather than being purged in the 1960s. Hence many TCM clinics offer qigong specialty clinics. Only after all other possibilities were exhausted did some families take their relatives to the psychiatric clinics.

At the very heart of this disorder was a central contradiction: how could a self-cultivation and healing practice lead to complications or even illness? Most people undertook qigong for its health benefits, not expecting the iatrogenic reactions more commonly associated with prescription medication. But although the majority of daily practitioners derived many positive health benefits from their efforts, some began to suffer in dramatic ways as a result of a lack of proper supervision or preconditioning. As mentioned in chapter 2, the proliferation of how-to manuals and the ease with which a person could attend mass qigong sessions by famous masters meant that large numbers of individuals could practice qigong on their own. For such people, their distress and dis-ease ironically stemmed from the sincere desire to heal themselves in the first place.

In this chapter I present two diverse contexts in which debates about qigong deviation took place. There was widespread conviction among biomedical professionals, qi masters, and laypeople that qigong was a powerful force capable of causing sickness, even mental illness. More than other forms of martial arts healing such as taiji, qigong was viewed as a potent technology of self-making and unmaking. While medical experts debated the etiology and cure for patients diagnosed with qigong deviation, qigong and martial arts practitioners viewed the phenomena from a different perspective, with their own conceptions about deviation in qigong practice and the necessary steps to alleviate distressing symptoms. TCM doctors were more likely to tell patients to discontinue qigong practice and use acupuncture and herbs to realign the qi. Beng-Yeong Ng summarized the way in which a TCM doctor might classify qigong deviation: sensory disturbances related to perceptions of abnormal qi flow, motor disturbances exhibited by uncontrollable or spasmodic movement stemming from qi blockages, or psychic disturbances such as altered consciousness, spirit possession, distracting thoughts, and mental derangement (1999, 200).

Family members were crucial navigators between the two competing systems of belief. Especially in a culture-bound disorder such as qigong deviation, before a person is brought to the psychiatric unit, family members have probably sought the services of traditional Chinese medicine practitioners, qigong masters, neighbors, friends, and colleagues. Such pluralistic approaches are usually not addressed in the literature on Chinese mental health care, where the focus is usually on institutional care or on social policy that addresses community resources. I hope to show how biomedical doctors interpreted the disorders and emerging symptoms associated with qigong. In doing so, I will examine why some people got institutionalized while others continued with daily practice. Scholars of classification practices have shown that normative behaviors are context specific (Bowker and Star 1999; Hacking 1998, 1999). Notions of what constitutes difference, or deviation, from norms are important sites for understanding the normative power of categories. In what follows, I juxtapose deviation in the two settings of qigong practice and psychiatric health care. My goal is to show how qigong deviation began as a manifestation of personal disorder and not as a disciplinary category by the state. By appropriating the indigenous classification system of deviation inherent within qigong practice, however, the state embarked on defining a different normative order.

DEVIATION IN CULTIVATION PRACTICES

Masters and long-term practitioners were aware of the existence of deviation in breathing exercises and self-cultivation practices long before the outbreaks of the 1990s. The indigenous phenomenon of deviation was referred to as *qigong piancha* (qigong deviation in lay terms) and sometimes *zouhuo rumo* (a classic Chinese phrase that translates as "leaving the path and demons entering"). To deviate (*zhou pian le*) or to leave the path meant several things: loss of balance and control over qi; inability to restore otherworldly visions or energy sensations to an ordinary context; and/or inappropriate practice or form. Zhouhuo rumo is a phenomenon found in martial art novellas and in cultivation practice. The term refers to becoming bewitched or possessed and losing control of one's faculties. Visions of deities, animals, or other natural forces are ordinary events in the practice of some martial art forms, particularly those with Daoist influences. For this reason, practitioners who experienced qigong deviation remained circumspect about their symptoms, seeking healers in confidence and keeping away from the asylum. Rather than being viewed as a psychiatric category of mental illness, the range of possible disorders involved in deviation was considered to be part of the long road to progress in one's practice. The popular image of qigong healing and masters in the public sphere supported this belief.

The many notions of deviation are evident in the richness of linguistic terms used to describe the phenomenon and accompanying experiences. A whole variety of terms describing loss of control fell into three categories: mechanical problems, sensory (primarily auditory and visual) problems, and possession. Phrases such as "I have deviated" (*wo pianle*) were used to describe the phenomenon.[1] The first category of mechanical problems was a common phenomenon that all practitioners faced initially during practice. After one first learned how to sense qi (both within and around oneself), the next step involved learning how to move qi throughout one's body. If the qi moved chaotically or moved suddenly to the head (similar to a phenomenon in kundalini yoga) during this step, it was necessary to focus on regaining the balance of elements in one's body.

Closely related to the first group of possible problems, the second category of deviation concerned sensory problems. As qigong practice opened the senses (*gongnengtong*) to the natural and supernatural worlds, it was not uncommon for individuals to hear voices of masters or alien entities communicating with them. Practitioners of specific forms often spoke of receiving external information or messages (*wai xin*) from other entities. Unwanted visions or hallucinations were also part of this stage. As one woman in her midfifties remarked, "I was terrified when I saw the tiger in the corner, but I closed my eyes and concentrated on my master's instructions and the image disappeared." Like the experience of qi movement in the body, visual and auditory perceptions were part of the ongoing process in everyday practice. Alleviation required strict discipline and working under the guidance of a master. At this stage, practitioners describe the extrasensory experiences as a challenge to overcome and a necessary threshold to higher levels of controlling the *qi* energy in one's body.

The third category of deviation, qigong possession, can be viewed as a continuum of diverse experiences ranging from simply being controlled by qi to total control by other entities (spiritual, animal, or human). Practitioners often referred to this phenomenon as zhouhuo rumo and considered the condition to be very serious, requiring expert help to resolve the problem. While the first two categories were considered to be a natural part of learning, this last category was viewed as an internal struggle with power. Learning to manage the boundaries between self and the external world was essential to achieving a balance of life forces within oneself.

Local means of intervention were syncretic, often including a mixture of methods taken from traditional Chinese medicine, Daoist healing, and folk tradition. As noted earlier, practitioners commonly sought the advice of the master from whom they had been taking instruction. For those who had learned from a popular publication instead of in the traditional way, seeking a healer involved an informal referral system by word of mouth or through the reference of masters. The 1980s saw a significant proliferation of qigong clinics at state institutions as well as the development of private specialists who focused on realigning the qi of wayward practitioners. Throughout the city streets were posters advertising private practices that involved qi healing for disorders ranging from simple ailments to more difficult cases (see fig. 11).

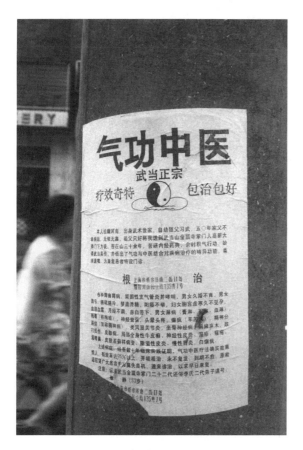

11. Street ad for a private qigong TCM clinic

Parallel to my clinical observations in the psychiatric ward, I also attended qigong healings of three types: traditional Chinese medical clinics that specialized in qigong treatment, private qigong clinics, and on-the-spot healing sessions. Most masters used the force of their qi to treat patients. In extreme cases of qigong possession, masters not only used qi healing but also incorporated Daoist exorcism practices. Master Ma, an older woman, practiced every day in Shanghai park. When I approached her, she playfully asked me how old I thought she was. I truthfully replied that she must be in her midfifties. As it turned out, Ma was in her midseventies and trained in qigong and traditional Chinese medicine by her father, who was a traditional healer. She was unusual because most traditional Chinese medical doctors (*lao zhongyi*) are male, as the knowledge of healing tends to descend along patrilineal lines. She operated a private clinic twice a week, on Thursday and Sunday afternoons, as a subcontractor to a traditional Chinese medicine hospital. When I attended the clinic, both old and new patients came to her for help. After diagnosing their ailments and giving herbal prescriptions, she would first massage the afflicted area and then focus on it with external *qi*. She occasionally encountered cases of mild deviation in which practitioners felt they lost control of their qi. Rather than feeling relaxed and healthy after practice, they found that the sensations of qi left them anxious and exhausted. Master Ma treated these instances of deviation primarily with traditional medicine such as acupuncture rather than with qigong.

I met Mr. Geng, a retired cadre and party member in his fifties, in the waiting room of another TCM qigong clinic in Shanghai. He had taken up qigong in 1978 for his neurasthenia. For the most part, his practice had beneficial effects, until he began to practice up to five or six hours per day without the supervision of a master. When he felt his qi move uncontrollably upward from his stomach to his head, Mr. Geng decided to seek help from Dr. Liu, a traditional medical doctor in Shanghai. He replied passionately when I asked what the experience of deviation felt like:

> No one knows how painful it is to deviate. The pain is indescribable. It's like dying and experiencing pain worse than death. No one understands this—not even the doctors or the masters. I often see qigong deviants with symptoms far milder than mine because my illness was so bad. I survived, but I know the pain. Qigong deviation is very different from mental illness, but, of course, there are some who are also mentally ill to begin with. Anyone who is recently upset or normally introverted shouldn't learn qigong.

The disorienting process of experiencing deep pain rather than relief described by Mr. Geng was not only mentally but also physically traumatic. Deviation in this case was far worse than the original illness that motivated him to start qigong practice in the first place.

Mr. Geng's cautious advice overlapped significantly with that of the majority of masters I interviewed on deviation. Master Lin, whose name card described him as a professor of medical qigong, believed that "learning too fast without good fundamentals" was the main cause. Master Chen, in his youthful thirties, believed that the mentally ill were more susceptible to deviation. Master Dong, in his sixties, listed three main causes: overdoing movements, overthinking during practice, and teaching oneself without a supervisor. He elaborated on the proper, or moral, ways to learn qigong. To cure deviation, he believed that a qigong master needed to act like a traditional doctor, considering diet and identifying appropriate methods for the particular individual. As a healer at the qigong association clinic, Master Cai had an even more specific response. Because there are many categories or forms of qigong, a person's constitution determined whether he or she was sensitive to qi. Once that has been established, the proper teacher made all the difference. Master Loo believed that having proper "posture, breath, and mindset" could effectively prevent deviation. My meeting with Master Liu, a female master in her fifties, led to a prophetic interview that foreshadowed the more orthodox view of deviation: "There are problems in the learning methods. It's important to use scientific methods and learn from a doctor or master. For too many years, our country was based on superstition. A lot of people are practicing and conducting research, but they've gone into a *kang* [battle] and don't even know it. If qigong continues to be a mess, we'll all be in a mess. Now qigong is a sham to get money." Her position reflected a stance that would be eventually taken up as state discourse on the practice. Such a range of responses indicates that masters were well aware of the phenomenon of deviation and had a variety of beliefs about its causation and treatment.

In the psychiatric context, patients who spoke of having the abilities to heal themselves or others were told by psychiatrists that they suffered from delusions. The official position on qigong healing, articulated clearly in state publications, was that such healing abilities involved suggestion (*ansi*) rather than scientific means of curing. The lay notion of healing could not be more different. In the everyday context, self-healing was both the means and the end. Behaviors that could be interpreted as deviation, such as unusual body movements and sounds, even trances, were considered a natural part of learning to align the rhythms of one's mind and body with the cosmos rather than remaining within the structures of official time and space. Warnings about deviation were a traditional part of learning qigong with a master. Even if one read about qigong and practiced without a master, it was still common knowledge that the practice required a peaceful environment and balanced emotions. Practitioners all repeated these conditions as necessary to their progress.

The phenomenon of spontaneous movement was a central to certain forms of qigong associated with deviation. Spontaneous movements included a range of uncharacteristic behaviors: individuals might cry or laugh, move freely, or remain quietly in trance. As Kenneth Cohen, an American teacher of qigong, writes, "In spontaneous qigong you are not moving the qi, the qi is moving you" (1997, 180). In the late 1980s and 1990s key sites for experiencing spontaneous movement were group practice in parks and mass qigong performances. In the parks, small groups gathered to practice in regular morning sessions.

It was not unusual to find people making animal-like gestures, running in place, or lying on the ground. It was primarily in the larger venues, however, that spontaneous movement was encouraged, to show the abilities of masters. A typical qigong performance could move audiences of several hundred, sometimes thousands, of people to simultaneous spontaneous movement. Hallways would be filled with loud groans, screams, burps, and clapping. It was not unusual to see individuals running up and down aisles patting themselves constantly on the head and body; others might move gracefully in movements evoking taiji. Such scenes reminded me of evangelical faith-healing sessions or rock concerts, occasions when individuals give themselves up to the rhythms and movements of energy within them.

The phenomenon of spontaneous movement raises key questions about boundaries and release. In his ethnographic research with practitioners of "cathartic qigong," Thomas Ots (1994) describes the trancelike state achieved in practice as a primary means to release and experience one's true self. In the context of the aftermath of Tiananmen and the eventual mobilization to the market economy, spontaneous movements were crucial forms of release from everyday life. After several months of interviews and observations, a regular group of practitioners I met with in the park encouraged me to try their form, which relied on spontaneous movements as part of their group healing practice. It was hard to shed my persona of social scientist at first, but an older woman placed her hands on my shoulders and told me, "You need to let go and just let yourself feel the qi." She then quickly twirled me around in small circles similar to the first movements of the game of pin-the-tail-on-the-donkey. With my eyes closed, I felt a sense of ease and floated to her encouragement. Peeking through one eye, I saw the dozen or so practitioners all had their hands pointed at me, making gestures of passing qi to me. When I regained my balance, the practitioners encouraged me to try again. Spontaneous movement was largely about letting go of inhibitions and allowing one's body to move without thinking.

In the world of qigong practitioners, deviation tended to be framed in terms of appropriateness of form and boundaries of knowledge. Deviation occurred when supervision was not adequate, the form was inappropriately matched to the practitioner, or the practitioner was not ready to progress to the next stage. Despite the possibilities of further, more serious consequences, qigong, self-cultivation, and healing forms continued to be popular. Notions of qi energy and the promise of being transformed by healing were found in diverse traditions, suggesting an interconnected web of meanings linking Chinese traditional medicine, martial arts, spiritual practice, and even contemporary science (especially physics and parapsychology).

In order to understand the reasons for qigong's popularity, it is important to look at the significance of miraculous healing in a social and political context devoted to modernization. The growth of qigong in urban China is intimately related to economic transformations that took place during the 1980s, even though the practice can be traced back to a long tradition of body practices. The popularity of qigong continued to expand because individual and social experiences of daily practice were generally beneficial. Qigong practitioners benefited from improved health and also reported having more harmonious family relations. Deviation, however, transformed initial pleasure and autonomy to discomfort and even excruciating pain, thus returning the individual to the familial and social matrix of order.

SPIRIT POSSESSION VERSUS POSSESSION BY QI

The practitioners of Great Universal qigong (*da zhiran gong*) continued to meet before the large tree in the park even after it was deemed to promote superstition. The widely popular but controversial master Xu was believed to have infused her special qi into the tree. Practitioners often sought it, claiming it had special healing powers. A regular group of twenty to thirty people went daily to engage in other realms of consciousness, focusing inward on their bodies and outward toward the universe. Many stood facing the tree with heads bowed in prayerlike positions or danced in circles twirling their hands and arms. A few lay on the ground in trance, sometimes moaning quietly. Others conversed in tongues (*yuzhouyu*), stopping at times to translate into Mandarin for me.

For those in the parks, possession was part of a larger continuum of practice. The trance state was both an ecstatic experience and a therapeutic process. A strong tradition of spontaneous movements can also be found in many martial art forms and in discussions of historic practices by cults such as the Boxers and White Lotus followers. In spite of being living in a socialist city facing the tremendous changes of modernization, practitioners could take pleasure in the sensual and cosmological world. Qigong practice transforms prescribed mentalities of urban living and allows one to navigate the chaos of everyday life with the power of self-healing. One could either give up control and succumb to the seductive power of qigong or slowly learn in moderation how to enhance one's health and longevity. The difficult process involved a delicate negotiation between ecstasy and pain. Possession and control by alien and spiritual entities through qigong practice was thus more commonly referred to as deviation (*chu pian* or zhouhuo rumo) rather than possession (*futi*) in Daoist terms.

The anthropological literature on possession provides critical comparative frameworks to assess the linkages between possession and marginality. Functional explanations, for instance—described extensively by I. M. Lewis (1989)—link possession primarily to powerlessness and the oppressed. Further anthropological studies that link possession and power consider possession to be both a temporal experience and gender specific in cross-cultural examples (Sharp 1993; Ong 1987). The ethnographic film *Les maîtres fous* (The mad masters), by Jean Rouch, helped me see how spiritual practices were experienced by the body and especially how possession can commence as a very physical and corporeal experience. Contemporary representations of possession in Western narrative films tend to emphasize the purely spiritual aspects of the experience, even as bodies are violently undone and remade. Though Rouch's film focuses on Hauka rituals by Nigerian migrant workers in post-colonial Ghana, the gestures, movements, and rituals particular to the post–World War II context shed light on the different states of trance and possession possible in qigong practice. One particular film sequence, where an initiate succumbs to possession initially in his right leg, helped to illuminate one practitioner's bewildering experience of feeling qi take over his leg and eventually his whole body.

Unlike other forms of possession, qigong possession was not gender specific: both males and females could become susceptible. Nor was the experience of qigong possession limited to the powerless: individuals from all social and political stations participated and sought healing from qigong. The experience of possession signaled that an individual had lost the power to negotiate and maintain a sense of control within him- or herself. Rather than becoming empowered through the experience of qigong possession, victims were viewed as disempowered, succumbing to chaos rather than achieving bodily and spiritual order through disciplined practice. Just as altered states can have multiple meanings, possession is an epiphenomenon that can be understood from different perspectives.

The activities in the park resembled the former pursuits described by institutionalized qigong patients. Those in the asylum had transgressed familial or social boundaries of normality such that confinement was necessary. In their experience, qigong possession was a psychiatric disorder that required drug therapy, rest, and the discontinuation of their practice. Normality meant overwhelming regularity and boredom in a daily routine of eating, sleeping, and eventually working.

The story of how qigong became an object of study in Chinese psychiatry reflects the power of medicalization to transform traditional notions of dis-ease and illness into biomedical categories of disease. Medicalization refers to the process of translating illness symptoms into medical categories.[2] Intersections between qigong and psychiatry did not begin as natural linkages on the part of practitioners in either field. Rather, as I will argue, the sum of key interventions such as institutional moves by state administrators to contain the popularity of certain qigong movements and the increased globalization of psychiatry led to the development of qigong deviation as a culture-bound disorder. Once created, this category nonetheless continued to coexist with different meanings in both the medical and the social realms. Understanding the consequences of this pathological category requires careful navigation between these vastly different frames of interpretation and through the range of experiences subsumed under the label of qigong deviation. The DSM-IV and Kenneth Cohen (1997) refer to this phenomenon as qigong psychosis. I prefer the local terms that were used during my field research. "Deviation" is a closer translation of the term *piancha* than is "psychosis." Other terms that have been used to refer to such symptoms include "cultivation insanity" and "martial arts madness."

In psychiatric clinical settings, qigong practitioners and patients described the experience of qigong deviation in two ways. The first category of symptoms related to mechanical problems with qi energy unleashed by qigong practice. In the outpatient clinic, patients described their difficulties to doctors who operated from a biomedical model of the body. Mr. Jiang, in his fifties, exclaimed, "Ever since I had problems concentrating, my qi has remained in my head, which is painful, so painful I want to kill myself." Another outpatient related how the qi in her stomach area could not be released, and consequently she had even greater difficulty with regular digestion and sleep. The second level of symptoms associated with qigong deviation involved uncontrollable visions and images with accompanying severe emotional distress, with great pain, anger, and fear. In some cases, simply attending a mass qigong session put individuals in a constant state of trance or distress for days afterward. One patient described being able to see and communicate with alien beings after his extrasensory perceptions opened with qigong (*gongneng tongle*) and the experience of seeing a famous master perform. The visions were welcomed at first, but soon he was unable to control when the aliens would contact him and occupy his mind and body. The descriptions of hallucinations and visions by qigong deviation patients overlapped with those of other mental patients, especially schizophrenics. Such overlap led many psychiatrists to question how to diagnose and treat patients whose symptoms corresponded with psychiatric categories.

QIGONG DISORDERS AS
CULTURE-BOUND SYNDROME

Culture-bound syndromes (CBS) are key areas where anthropological knowledge offers much insight for psychiatric practice. The term refers to specific illness categories that tend to be associated with particular cultures and groups of people. For instance, syndromes such as *amok* in Southeast Asian and *nervios* in Latin American societies are widely known outside the psychiatric setting. The Diagnostic and Statistical Manual of Mental Disorders (DSM) is the set of classification codes for the diagnosis of psychiatric disorders used in most contemporary practices in addition to the International Classification of Disorders (ICD). In the DSM-IV, there were several additions, including an appendix that outlined steps for the clinical formulation of culture-bound syndromes of twenty-five recognized phenomena. The growing recognition of culture-bound syndromes is reflected in the increased number of categories with each revision of the DSM.

Such professional acknowledgment of new categories is related to the increasingly visible role culture plays in psychiatry (Johnson 1988). Three categories were associated with Chinese culture: *shenjing shuairuo* (neurasthenia), *shenkui* (a mix of depression, neuroses, and anxiety), and qigong psychotic reaction. In one sense, the inclusion of these categories indicates a grudging acknowledgment of culture in the experiences of mental illness and the need for tools that can assess mental and social disorders according to different cultural contexts within psychiatry.[3] These categories also reflect processes of diagnosis based on shared meanings among professionals around the globe. The implementation of uniform practices such as codes from the DSM-IV reflects a growing acceptance of the equivalence necessary to globalize discourses such as psychiatry. The development of mutually constitutive categories in this discipline reveals how globalization is not just about material goods and cultural symbols for consumption in local contexts. Officially recognized terms of illness and forms of mental health care indicate that globalization is also about the implementation of normative practices at mundane, everyday levels.

Shenjing shuairuo, the clinical diagnosis given for the experience of weak nerves, fatigue, sleeplessness, headache, dizziness, and other complaints, remains one of the most widely recognized and diagnosed categories in Chinese psychiatric clinics today. Causal explanations for this category stem from Soviet theories in which unfavorable conditions cause tensions in the nervous system, thus weakening a person's constitution. In tracing the usage and eventual demise of the diagnosis of neurasthenia in the United States, Arthur Kleinman (1986) asserted that the continued diagnosis of this disorder rather than clinical depression in China reflected much about the cultural meanings of somatization. At present, "neurasthenia" continues to be used as an equivalent translation for shenjing shuairuo, even though the frequency of this diagnosis has decreased considerably in recent years.

In a collection of essays in the journal *Culture, Medicine, Psychiatry*, Chinese practitioners and scholars argued for the necessity of retaining neurasthenia as a diagnostic concept in China (Yan 1989; Lee 1999). While Western psychiatrists might diagnose such symptoms as depression, Chinese professionals argued that the category was still prominent in Chinese culture and hence a critical code. The call to retain neurasthenia as an indigenized category reflected an ongoing concern with the high presence of sufferers both in clinics and elsewhere. Literary explorations of this condition during the May Fourth movement as well as contemporary social discourses indicate that as a cultural category, neurasthenia remained a powerful signifier of the absence of agency both at the individual level and for the body politic. Debates about neurasthenia and shenjing shuairuo illustrate how, even with shared diagnostic categories, the use of these codes and the professional meanings of such symptoms are nonetheless embedded in cultural contexts. Psychiatry might be a globalizing discourse, but the translation or translatability of symptoms is highly dependent on the professionals who use them and the everyday contexts that encompass their meanings.

Whereas shenjing shuairuo stems from a specific relationship with an environment of social stress, the category of qigong psychotic reaction is related to a healing practice. The DSM-IV includes the following definition of this phenomenon: "A term describing an acute, time-limited episode characterized by dissociative, paranoid, or other psychotic or nonpsychotic symptoms that may occur after participation in the Chinese folk health enhancing practice of qigong ('exercise of vital energy'). Especially vulnerable are individuals who become overly involved in the practice. This diagnosis is included in the *Chinese Classification of Mental Disorders*, Second Edition (CCDM-2)" (1994, 847).

The CCDM is another diagnostic handbook with a history worth noting. The first version was published in 1983, after a conference of psychiatrists. In his introduction, Dr. Derson Young acknowledged the need for a manual intended for Chinese professionals. Compiling the manual involved not only the translation of categories recognized in the DSM-III but also the inclusion of categories such as neurasthenia not acknowledged outside China but deemed important for use there. The third edition of CCDM was released in April 2002 in both Chinese and English. The second edition organized qigong deviation into two categories: (59.1) *qigong suozhi jingshen zhangai* (psychosis made by qigong) and (59.2) *qigong youfa jingshen zhangai* (psychosis induced or related to qigong). Though the two categories were nearly identical, the first category considered criteria such as "qigong, hypnosis, meditation, yoga, and autogenic training" to be causative of psychosis, while the second considered factors such as "*mixin* (superstition) and *wushu* (wizardry)" to exacerbate existing mental illness (Chinese Medical Association 1990, 66–67). In other words, the first group mainly addressed those individuals who had never experienced mental disorders before learning qigong, while the second grouped together already mentally unstable people with the predisposition to deviation. Most Chinese psychiatrists continue to refer to the phenomenon in lay terms as qigong deviation (*qigong piancha*). Only occasionally, in cases where the patient's behavior warranted the term, did psychiatrists ever invoke the specific term "qigong-induced psychosis" (*qigong suozhi jingshen zhangai*).

All the qigong deviation patients (there were at least three or four—over 6 percent—in each inpatient ward) distinguished themselves from the general patient population in terms of their state of affect, which seemed quite functional; most patients good-naturedly engaged in animated conversations with me. Like patients diagnosed with depression or psychosomatic disorders, they tended not to think of themselves as mentally ill and felt that they did not belong in the wards. While they stood out in appearance and manner at first, gradually the rhythm of ward life anesthetized them to a daily routine of structured activity, drug therapy, and sleep.

In the team meeting held once a week, two new cases were chosen for discussion and teaching purposes during my first rotation in the wards. Both cases involved qigong deviation. The head doctor of the second-floor ward and the head nurse led the discussion. "There have already been three patients admitted since January, and now there are two more." The team reviewed the occupied hospital beds to see who could be released so that new patients could be admitted. The focus of the rehabilitation team was to get patients through the program, to encourage progress rather than to punish. The attending team of doctor and nurses spent much time on behavior modification within the hospital, monitoring responses to medication and feedback from family members. The team meeting was remarkable in that the health care workers were divided as to how to distinguish true sufferers of qigong deviation from schizophrenics who also happened to practice qigong. In the discussion that followed, one senior psychiatrist noted that in a sample study of one hundred patients in Shanghai with qigong-related disorders, 80 percent were male and 20 percent female. In contrast, many of the patients admitted for deviation in Beijing were female. All the patients had no previous history of mental illness. After practicing qigong, however, all claimed to be able to visualize illness within the body and to be able to cure others with this power. While the younger residents—in their thirties and forties—expressed the belief that the phenomenon was a culture-specific disorder (or culture-bound syndrome), an older generation of psychiatrists (in their sixties), now in official hospital positions, voiced caution and argued for maintaining the category of schizophrenia. It was apparent that many psychiatric workers were unfamiliar with the disorder and wished to be judicious about diagnosis and treatment until a clear pattern emerged.

Initially, most psychiatrists were reluctant to label the disorder with the new category. Instead, patients were admitted with the initial diagnoses of schizophrenia, hysteria, or other mental illnesses until further observation and response to drug therapy could be obtained. In addition, many of the initial disorders associated with qigong deviation were similar to panic attacks, in which individuals experienced hyperventilation, rapid elevation of pulse, dizziness, and great anxiety over spontaneous movements. This process of wait and see acknowledges the overlap and sometimes indistinguishable characteristics of qigong deviation and other mental illnesses—chiefly anxiety and delusions.

Interviews with patients and family members as well as participant observation with clinicians made me recognize the need to compare the experience of inpatients with those who went to the outpatient clinics with qigong-related disorders. The situation of qigong patients in a psychiatric clinic setting seemed odd, especially since the individual patients did not consider themselves to be mentally ill. Yet this was overridden by family members, who thought the experiences of zouhuo rumo (qigong possession) warranted an exam by a psychiatrist. Similar to patients diagnosed with depression or psychosomatic disorders, qigong deviation patients felt that they did not belong in the psychiatric wards. By the time a person was admitted into the ward, mental distress was so advanced that qigong-induced mental disorder or psychotic reaction (*qigong suozhi jingshen zhangai*) was no longer the primary disorder. Rather, this diagnosis seemed to be applicable for a specific and limited time to patients whose behavior returned to normal once practice was discontinued. Those individuals who continued to be unmanageable and have hallucinations or delusions tended to be classified as schizophrenic or suffering from reactive psychosis. The psychiatric community throughout China was reluctant to adopt the new category unless patient symptoms clearly corresponded with the Chinese classification. The tenuousness of the category is also due to the possibility that many patients themselves were either mentally ill before taking up the practice or, more likely, reluctant to perceive their condition as a mental disorder.

QIGONG DEVIATION
IN SHANGHAI

In April 1990, after three months of observation and inter-
views of mental patients in Beijing, I left for Shanghai to attend a nationwide
psychiatric workshop, "The Treatment and Rehabilitation of Chronic
Mentally Ill," sponsored by the World Health Organization (WHO) and the
World Association for Psychiatric Rehabilitation (WAPR). The director of my
institute was to be a major discussant as the head of a primary WHO center
for mental health rehabilitation and research. The conference was held at the
Shanghai Mental Health Center with participants (mainly directors or vice-
directors) representing psychiatric institutes from all over China. It was by
pure coincidence that I met Dr. Guo, one of the earliest psychiatrists to conduct research on the disorder termed qigong deviation.

On the morning of April 23, 1990, I rode my bicycle to the Shanghai Mental Health Center, which, ironically, happened to be next door to the Shanghai
Qigong Institute. Like any visitor, I had to show my identity card at the gate
and state my reasons for entering the compound. After signing in, I ran to the
main lecture hall, where the opening speeches had already begun. The audience
was filled with a mix of psychiatrists in everyday clothes and those from the host
institute in white hospital coats. Giant red banners announcing the title of the
conference hung at the front of the room over the main table where hosts, officials, and visiting WHO experts sat. I took a seat in the back next to a local doctor. As the speeches proceeded, I asked this neighbor to help identify each participant. We introduced ourselves and asked each other about research interests.
I mentioned my interest in qigong deviation. He replied enthusiastically, "Perhaps this is fate. I published the first psychiatric article on qigong deviation."
The rest of the speeches droned on in the background as we continued our animated discussion. My mind was filled with questions, which I later asked.
What do you think about this disorder? Why is it called "deviation"? Do you
see any epidemiological patterns of status, age, gender, or physical conditions?
Are there any regional differences? How do you treat patient symptoms? What
about family members—is there any correlation between family (non)support
and manifestations? Are you still working with these patients? As the morning
ceremony drew to a close, Dr. Guo and I arranged to meet again for a detailed
discussion of his work and to interview several of his patients.

The rest of the weeklong conference consisted of WHO lectures, special pre-
sentations of regional programs, tours of Shanghai rehabilitation centers, visits
to factories (with patient employees), and conference discussion groups. The
participants' commitment to patient care and reviewing existing services was

evident. Discussions about regional difference, epidemiology, social support networks, and modes of intervention were often heated. The majority (over 80 percent) of chronic patients treated in rehabilitation programs throughout China were diagnosed as schizophrenic, institutionalized on average for over ten years or more. When I inquired about qigong patients, the response by these colleagues was that only a handful of such cases ever made it to the inpatient wards as chronic cases. The phenomenon seemed to be primarily confined to urban regions, and most cases were dealt with in outpatient wards. These observations by psychiatrists from provinces throughout China coincided with Dr. Guo's initial findings.

In our meeting several days later, Dr. Guo outlined his experience with the phenomenon of qigong deviation. The following summarizes his account:

> In 1984, when I was on a clinical psychiatry rotation, I noticed a number of patients who all claimed the cause of their mental disorder was their qigong practice. I found that most of these patients were not psychotic but seemed to exhibit a new category of a culture-bound syndrome. I started collecting medical histories mainly from outpatient clinics and outlining the clinical phenomenology. As it turned out, the Shanghai Qigong Association next door has a special department devoted to qigong deviation. My interest in this work also grew when a famous master started to become quite fashionable in China. The popularity of qigong in China is a new mental health issue. Recently, so many people are returning to the temples as part of a general rise in religious activity. There needs to be so much more research carried out on this topic; there ought to be studies on stigma, rating scales of depression and neurosis, community outreach programs, comparative data between family members of schizophrenic patients and qigong patients, control studies of psychology, even transcultural comparisons. The relation with traditional Chinese medicine needs to be understood. We also need a comparative study of normal people who practice and these psychiatric patients. So far the pattern seems to indicate three areas of difference: emotional disturbance, uncontrollable practice, and susceptibility to neurosis. Dr. Young [the director of psychiatry in central China] happens to believe that this is a very important problem. That is why my findings were published in the Chinese Classification and Diagnostic Manual in 1989.

I found out that the term "deviation" was chosen in English because it was equivalent to the lay term *piancha.*

During the rest of my stay in Shanghai, I was able to meet several of Dr. Guo's patients who were willing to talk about their experiences. The first patient that he introduced, Tong, was a twenty-nine-year-old high school graduate who had been a factory worker for over ten years. He started learning sanyuancheng qigong in 1981 to improve his physical ability. Now he is not allowed to practice anymore and is presently taking chlorpromazine (150 milligrams a day). When I asked how he came to be at the hospital, he replied,

> One night as I was practicing my father yelled suddenly, which scared me, so I hid under the bed. I am used to noise at home since there are five of us still (two older siblings have moved away already). I have never been afraid of my father, but I always argue with my mother. The old man reported my behavior to the factory because I would not let him sleep at night. I like qigong because it makes me feel good, but I will not practice anymore because I have been in here [the ward] too long. I could cure people for things such as sore backs. I realized I had a problem when I came to the hospital; no one understands me except the doctors. After I leave this place, I will continue painting as a hobby.

After Tong returned to the other side of the locked ward, Dr. Guo gave further background about this patient. In early June 1989, he was reported by a factory official for his disruptive behavior at home and at work. One midnight, Tong suddenly sat upright and cried, "My father has died!" He ran to the factory, but, finding the door closed, he then ran to the home of his master. Tong promptly tore off all his clothes and went to sleep on the old man's bed. He believed that a force was controlling him. At the initial outpatient exam, he was extremely violent and unwilling to cooperate. Afraid of being hospitalized, he ran away after the exam to a friend in Shandong Province (neighboring Shanghai). After his money ran out, Tong returned to the factory and hid out until payday. When he went to collect his wages, the work unit brought him to the hospital to check in as an inpatient. It was at this time that his initial diagnosis of qigong deviation was changed to schizophrenia as the primary condition. The narratives of the work unit and family were viewed by physicians as legitimate.

The second patient, Ling, was a twenty-eight-year-old college-educated engineer who was very far away from his work unit in Ningbo, Gansu Province. After a bout with hepatitis in 1988, he started qigong in December 1989 to cure himself. His teacher was one of his coworkers in the work unit and had cured cases of cancer. Ling believed he was making progress until he started yelling and screaming uncontrollably. He was quick to point out to me the link between his emotional distress and the problems he experienced. "The reason I am such trouble is that I learned qigong when I was upset. In 1988 I was engaged, but since I did not recover from hepatitis, my fiancée left me. Qigong moves the emotions [*qigong dong ganqing*]. People with unsteady emotions should not learn qigong. I was sent here by my work unit, and I have been here for two and a half months now. I am staying here for hepatitis and not as a qigong patient." It is useful to note that in TCM, the liver is the seat of emotions. Ling's attempt to practice qigong to alleviate hepatitis and his emotional stress backfired. In his mind, qigong deviation was not the primary cause but a secondary outcome of his earlier physical problems with his liver.

When I inquired about his practice, Ling quickly replied, "I still have qi. I learned with a coworker, and we have the same qi. It's possible to pass along our qi and even our thoughts." He continued to talk about qigong enthusiastically. "There is definitely a presence in qigong. For example, living things such as trees have qi that is related to the energy in our liver. We need the qi of trees just as the tree needs our qi. It is better to practice outside where the air is better. It is possible to make predictions of the future or have sudden flashes of knowledge if you are sensitive [*ling gan*]."

His conversation suddenly shifted to his personal relations and the incidents that led to his hospitalization.

My relationship with my brother is quite friendly. My family thinks something is wrong and that I am mentally ill, but my friends do not really know about my illness. In January 1990, after learning qigong for a month, I still felt upset, especially by other people. I could sense their impressions of me, and so I would go up to them and be quite rude. The night before I came here, I went to my girlfriend's home to clear things up. Afterward I fought with someone on the streets, and my abilities were lost. I still believe in qigong, and after I leave I intend to continue learning. Qigong is definitely related to Buddhism, and now I am Buddhist. I have more insight about myself and humanity.

Ling closed his eyes for a moment and ended, "To be a human one must act as a balanced person." After Ling left, I was informed by an attending nurse that his primary diagnosis was no longer qigong deviation but reactive psychosis.

THE BEIJING QIGONG CLINIC

In May 1990, a devoted psychiatrist who was also intrigued by the phenomenon of qigong deviation opened the first specialized psychiatric outpatient clinic in Beijing devoted to this disorder. Though the initial number of cases was not large, each week brought more patients who had learned of the clinic by word of mouth, referral, or newspaper reports. Dr. Lin, a tall woman in her forties, was the director of the first team meeting to discuss qigong inpatient cases that I attended. Being a qigong practitioner initially, she was intrigued by the outbreak of patients and decided to transfer to the outpatient clinics. At first, her responsibilities only allowed her to conduct a special psychiatric clinic once a week, on Tuesday afternoons. Former inpatients were required to return to the clinic for follow-up care within a few weeks of their discharge. Most qigong patients were then directed to Dr. Lin's clinic. Whereas previously I had rotated from clinic to clinic to become acquainted with different psychiatric specialties, the Tuesday qigong clinic became a regular part of my participant observation.

Dr. Lin's credibility as both psychiatrist and practitioner initially raised questions for other staff members. Once, in the hallway, she was taken aside by the head nurse, a senior psychiatrist, and a handful of younger doctors who asked her whether or not qi was a "true" phenomenon that she personally experienced. She responded, "Yes, we all have qi. You can feel it between your own hands if you slowly pull them apart and then put them together. Gradually you will feel a small ball of energy that goes from your hands to circulate within your body." Dr. Lin gradually started to sway from side to side in trancelike motions. A few of the younger residents tried to imitate Dr. Lin's gestures, while the older psychiatrist and head nurse looked unconvinced. As an observer, I realized that Dr. Lin's view of the disorder as a believer would be transformed.

In the clinics, some of the individuals recognized me from the inpatient wards. Yet each week I saw a wide range of patients who never made it into the wards. While most of the qigong inpatients had overlapping diagnoses of schizophrenia or other disorders and were undergoing psychopharmacological treatment, many of the outpatients presented different symptoms. One patient had traveled all the way from Xian City (over an eight-hour train journey) to see Dr. Lin. As he waited in the hallway, he suddenly started coughing and gasping for breath in uncontrollable spasms that made him double over. Between gasps he told me that the qi in his body would not stop circulating and the malady interfered with his regular breathing. Dr. Lin recorded the patient's medical history as well as his account of qigong practice and then told him that the symptoms were psychosomatic and could be cured. The news calmed the outpatient momentarily before another spasm started.

I traveled to Shanghai and Shandong Province during the summer months to conduct comparative regional studies of rural mental health care programs and qigong deviation. On my return to Beijing in September 1990, Dr. Lin's specialty clinic had expanded to Tuesday and Thursday afternoons. There was also a noticeable difference in her approach to practice. After a hectic afternoon of seeing patients, she confided that she had attended a special conference on qigong sponsored by the Ministry of Health at Beidaihe (a summer resort). "My understanding about qigong is very different. Now I realize that much of my belief in qigong and the sensations of qi [*qi gan*] was mainly due to self-suggestion [*ziwo ansi*]. This is the case for many qigong patients as well. They have delusions that qigong can cure anything and that they have qi inside themselves. I am now using the suggestion of qi to help cure these patients." Dr. Lin proudly pulled out from her desk several articles that had been published in the *Jiankang Ribao* (Health daily). "I wrote these after my participation in the conference, and I am looking forward to writing a book about this phenomenon." It was apparent that Dr. Lin had evolved from being a participant to the more public state role of health educator. Her conversion from clinical doctor to one of the leading specialists of the emerging disorder also meant a more public role in which she was called upon to speak about the disorder as a state figure.

The rhythm of the outpatient clinics is much more hectic than that of the wards, with their prescribed tranquillity and rest cure. Dr. Lin's clinic was busiest during the afternoons. An average psychiatrist may see six or seven patients during a four-hour shift; during April and May Dr. Lin saw eight to ten (sometimes twelve). Several months later the outpatients dwindled to six patients per afternoon clinic. During my participation, from May 1990 to January 1991, I observed a total of one hundred and fifteen patients. This figure does not represent the total number of qigong patients; there were many clinics I was unable to attend because of scheduling.

The stories of the outpatients varied greatly, as many had different backgrounds, but there were several common themes. First, all patients sought qigong as a form of healing for chronic ailments. After trying many other options, including Western medicine and traditional Chinese medicine, they turned to qigong as an alternative healing practice. Second, after beginning to practice, most patients initially sensed immense qi energy in their bodies but later were unable to control its direction. This led to actions such as running out into the street at night to alleviate sensations of heat and overpowering energy. Finally, another common pattern of patients in the psychiatric clinic was the experience of being especially sensitive to sounds or natural phenomena such as light or heat. These patients later were categorized as delusional. As with other outpatients, most qigong deviation patients came to the clinic as a result of the efforts of their families. Family members turned to the clinic when they could no longer cope with the unpredictability of the disorder on their own.

My ten-day absence from the wards during the conference was noted by the inpatients. When I returned to visit the women's ward, the younger patients in the recreation room called out "Nancy!" and told me about their progress and changes in my absence. Most of the patients had gained weight, an average of eight *jin* (about ten pounds). After I finished greeting the women on the second-floor ward, I walked downstairs to the courtyard, where male patients were walking outdoors. Several were playing basketball, while others strolled clockwise around the perimeter of the garden. There were several new inpatients, but I did not introduce myself right away. Instead, I was mesmerized by the sight of a group of five patients gathered in a corner standing silently together around the single tree in the yard with their heads cocked to the right side. "What are they doing?" I asked another patient standing nearby. "Oh, they are just practicing qigong together," the woman replied. I was stunned. I had assumed that once people were admitted as inpatients, they would no longer continue with their practice. It was actively discouraged, and family members were instructed by psychiatrists to prevent patients from any contact with practitioners or qigong literature. Yet in the enclosed environment of the asylum during the recreation hour, when only a handful of staff workers could preside, a few enthusiasts gathered to practice in quiet communion, momentarily away from the watchful eyes of family, work unit, or state institutions.

As I watched, the group members suddenly broke into quick individual movements. Each person gracefully swayed from side to side, moving hands up and down, dancing or moving with taiji martial arts movements. They seemed indifferent to other patients, and yet sometimes one would stop to place a hand two inches over the *dantian* (acupuncture point at lower abdomen) of another patient, presumably to heal an ailment. The practitioners seemed to move in another realm of consciousness and yet could return to the present moment easily.

One practitioner came toward me and asked how I was doing. I had a number of questions but only asked, "What were you doing as a group before you broke apart?" The patient smiled, "We were absorbing external information from our master" (*women zai shou waixin cong laoshi*). I was transfixed because at last I could see the transformative phenomenon of qigong practice by individuals, who in spite of being hospitalized and treated with psychotropic drugs, managed to find moments of consciousness and alignment with an external world beyond the walls of the asylum and the state.

QIGONG DEVIATION NARRATIVES

In *Qigong Chupian* (Qigong emergent deviation), Dr. Zhang Tongling (1997) began with an analysis of the category before presenting forty medical histories. Narratives such as "A Mother's Tears" and "Mother and

Daughter Both Ill" indicated the desperate plight that many of the patients and their families faced. The work was based on 356 clinical cases seen over an eight-year period, from 1983 to 1991, with slightly more female patients (56.2 percent) and an average age of thirty-nine-and-a-half years, ranging from fourteen to seventy-three. Cadres constituted the biggest group of qigong deviation patients (41.3 percent); workers accounted for 36.8 percent, students for 14.3 percent, domestic workers for 2.5 percent, farmers for 2.2 percent, and others for 2.9 percent. In following CCDM criteria, Dr. Zhang found a slight majority of patients (53.75 percent) in the first category of qigong-induced psychosis (*qigong suozhi jingshen zhangai*) than in the second group of psychosis exacerbated by qigong (*qigong youfa jingshen zhangai*). She also elaborated on the main symptoms to be found in these groups, including hallucinations (*huanjue*), paranoia (*wanxiang*), and anxiety (*jiaolu*). In addition to Zhang's comprehensive study, another carried out by C. M. Han and W. J. Ji, also in Beijing, with 479 qigong patients, had very similar findings (Ng 1999, 201).

The appearance of qigong deviation as a psychiatric diagnostic category, its associated behaviors and dramatic symptoms, and the narratives of experiences by patients and family members are a window onto the cultural anxieties and concerns that mostly urban residents faced in the 1990s. While the stories of the patients and families are quite different, they face similar challenges in seeking care. Encounters with the mental health care system involved constant negotiation for diagnosis, treatment, and attention by staff. Particularly for those patients diagnosed with the emergent category of qigong deviation in the early 1990s, the intervention and involvement of family members were crucial not only for the eventual recovery of the patient but also for the proper institutional responses of hospital staff, work units, neighbors, and even public security. Inside the psychiatric wards, relatives frequently discussed drug regimens and diagnostic categories with staff while trying to relate to their family members and update them with news of recent events in their lives. In the outpatient clinics, there was a continuous search for the elusive diagnosis. In the everyday realm, the family had to pick up the pieces and return to routines disrupted by sudden incidents of madness or frequent visits to the mental health center.

Recent studies of Chinese families that live with long-term mental disorders such as chronic schizophrenia have focused on the coping strategies that evolved in response to the tremendous social and economic changes in the PRC since the mid-1980s (Phillips 1998; Pearson and Phillips 1994). These studies include collaborative quantitative and qualitative research with Chinese colleagues that shows the ways in which the socioeconomic resources of a family may determine the long-term access and care that a patient receives. From their study of memory, experiences of alienation, and somatized pain of the Cultural Revolution, Joan and Arthur Kleinman point out how individual experiences are based in "local, moral worlds" that are shaped by families and work units (1999:20). In Chinese society, the social unit, especially the family, bears the responsibility of management and care for individuals suffering from mental illness. Moreover, family members are not only implicated in daily care and routines of assistance but often responsible for any legal matters and for negotiating with work units or hospitals for their relatives' well-being (Phillips et al. 2000).

Here, I supplement illness narratives with stories from the family members who were intimately involved in the caretaking, advocacy, and administration of health care. Like life histories, such narratives offer insight into the daily struggles with disease and medical institutions. When contextualized within larger frames of historic changes and political economy, they can also illuminate the agency or powerlessness that individuals face within hegemonic institutions. The stories reframe both medical histories, which tend to offer cases from the perspective of the medical institution, and patient narratives, which only focus on individuals. Furthermore, such narratives offer ways to understand the social dimensions of suffering rather than focusing solely on pathological accounts of an individual patient. As mentioned earlier, many literate patients in urban clinics often brought in their own written medical narratives to offer as the medical record. Similar clinical encounters have been described in ethnographic accounts by medical anthropologists Judith Farquhar (1994) and Arthur Kleinman (1986).

The following four stories explore how differently the emerging disorder was experienced and the dilemmas of being placed in a new psychiatric category. Initially, most psychiatrists were reluctant to label the disorder with the new category. Instead, patients were admitted with an early diagnosis of schizophrenia until further observation and response to drug therapy could be obtained. This process acknowledges the overlapping and sometimes indistinguishable characteristics of qigong deviation and schizophrenia—chiefly hallucinations and delusions.

After my first month of observing and interviewing in the wards, most staff members knew that I was interested in any incoming qigong cases. In late January, I was alerted that a new patient had been admitted into the male ward. I missed meeting the family during routine admission procedures, but the patient was already in the dining area. He sat on a bench with legs crossed, constantly hitting himself and repeating his name over and over again. Sometimes he rocked back and forth. My initial meeting with Zhong was difficult; often, he appeared to zone out into another realm. Later interviews became much easier, as he could carry on a long conversation and give descriptions of his experience. He would tell his story punctuated with small nervous laughs.

Zhong was classified as schizophrenic. In addition, while other patients were brought in by family members, he had been released from the local jail for psychiatric observation as his behavior was considered abnormal. His case illustrated a peculiar series of intersections among mental illness, the impact of the Tiananmen demonstrations, and qigong deviation. According to his father, during the months of April, May, and June 1989, Zhong went to Tiananmen to observe and participate in the growing demonstrations. Immediately after the crackdown, his father sent him to his grandparents' home in rural Jiangsu Province. In the fall, Zhong ran away to Shanghai to attend courses at the local medical college. When he was unable to present proper identification when challenged, university security sent him to the Shanghai police, who promptly transferred him back to Beijing from the Shanghai jail. It was during this period in the Beijing prison that he returned to his former practice of qigong. Time stood still, and the monotonous routine of being fed *wotou* (a type of coarse cornmeal) twice a day only made him more determined to escape. When I asked about this experience, he responded, "There were others [about twenty inside the cell] who knew how to practice qigong, and we started talking about different *gongfa* [methods]. So I started practicing again. Soon I would heal people with my qi. Now I am a true master with *teyigongneng* [paranormal abilities]."

In the medical history, Zhong was described as introverted and rather inhibited (*neixiang, danxin*). There had been no history of mental illness in his family for two generations. The diagnosis of schizophrenia as the primary condition was unique, as Zhong was very involved with qigong. According to the attending nurses and physicians, he still had delusions of thinking of himself as a master. Remarks such as, "I have come to the mental hospital to study qigong and see how I can cure people" or "I have teyigongneng and do not need to eat or sleep" were noted in his history as evidence of such delusions.

On family visiting days, Zhong's father came regularly. As an intellectual, he viewed his son's bout of mental illness and unmanageability as a result of pressures from the crackdown after June 4th. His mother attended Sunday visit days and was eager to draw her son from his shell. She brought his favorite noodles each week along with several *jin* of seasonal fruit. Both parents were very open to my questions and wished to fill in gaps in the medical record whenever possible. As Zhong's stay in the ward progressed, his hyperactive energy subsided, and he became more calm, even gaining twenty pounds.

With her habit of tossing her head defiantly and her steady gaze, Li stood out from the other patients. She and the other qigong patients did not consistently follow the pattern of the other mental health care program. Compliance with a therapeutic program meant taking prescribed psychotropic drugs, eating three meals a day, and sleeping endlessly. While they were made to adhere to this regimen, the the qigong patients continued the rhythms of their practice even inside the ward.

Beliefs about becoming a master or having intimate relationships with masters were frequently articulated by qigong patients. While Zhong reported having delusions of being a master, Li believed that she was to marry her master. Like Zhong she reported having teyigongneng after practicing healing for two months. She believed her powers gave her the ability to heal others, especially after she began to feel qi all over her body and to see colors in other people. The voice of Li's master stayed with her when she was first admitted to the inpatient ward. "Don't take these medicines. Qigong can cure you still. Just listen to me and keep practicing." As the other patients paced from room to room, walking off the effects of the drugs, she sat in lotus position, concentrating on her breath imagery. Occasionally she would rise from her position to join others for meals. With contact mostly limited to the ritual checkup each morning, staff members were unaware of her private practice.

The eldest sister's account gave more specific examples of how Li's transformation had made her more recalcitrant at home. She started breaking glass and tearing off her clothes. The family took Li to Huilongguan Hospital, a larger municipal mental hospital on the outskirts of Beijing, where she was diagnosed with schizophrenia. Her family then sought further expertise from the Institute of Mental Health, because they believed the medication prescribed for Li was not very effective. She felt much more positive about being at a research hospital that was focused more on short-term stays and research than long-term stays.

As mentioned earlier, Li stood out for her proud stance and active engagement with hospital staff where other patients quietly watched. Such actions sometimes got her into trouble, however, when they were characterized as violent. At times, she felt controlled by external entities, and this led to her being sedated or put in semiisolation from the other patients. After ninety-eight days of hospitalization Li was discharged from the hospital but was resigned to staying at home with light housework. Her job at the biscuit factory was no longer available. She did not practice qigong anymore.

Downstairs on the men's ward, Chen was plagued by instructions in an alien "universal" language (yuzhouyu). He was accompanied by his wife, who was allowed to stay through special arrangement with the hospital. (In cases where acute care was needed—for example, physical conditions and violent cases—permission was given for family members to stay with the patient so that twenty-four-hour attendance could be given without additional staffing.) Chen's wife, Wang, drew attention, especially in the all-male ward. The other females present in the men's ward were hospital staff—nurses, cleaners, or doctors. I approached Wang, an intensely earnest middle-aged woman, after first indicating that I was not a doctor but a research scholar interested in family roles in the management of mental illness. She mentioned that her husband was seeking care for qigong deviation but quickly admitted, "It's ironic, but if anyone should be here, it should be myself."

I quickly blurted, "Why?" She continued:

Because I was the one learning qigong in the first place. I have chronic digestive problems, and I started practicing last year. My husband started to accompany me because it was a long way to the park. He made progress more quickly than I did, but soon he could not control himself anymore. He started to practice four to five hours a day and then started to hear and see things. He received external messages [*waixin*] to kill himself, but he did not want to and was terrified of doing anything more.

The sensation of losing control and instead being moved by an external power was shared by many qigong patients. Mr. Gao, a male patient in his fifties, described how his practice of Daoist qigong progressed as expected until one day the qi in his right leg became "stuck." "I was walking along Wangfujing Street and suddenly felt as if my right leg had a will of its own. I started walking in a wide circle, because the leg became planted on the ground and my other leg tried to continue going forward. I had to stop and really concentrate before my leg could move again." I asked how he came to be in the ward. He continued, "Well, it was either the ward or jail." My eyebrows raised.

I was walking down the street several days ago, and the same problem happened. I first lost control of one leg and then the other soon after. No concentration on controlling this force could help. My legs started walking without my control, and I started grabbing signposts and people to try to stay in one place. But to no avail: my legs were taking me toward Tiananmen Square. I called out to the soldiers not to shoot, as I could not help myself. They leveled their arms at me, but I managed to convince them I needed help, so here I am.

At the time, we both giggled nervously at hearing such an unbelievable tale. Before hearing Gao's story, I found it hard to imagine how a person—or a body part, in this case—could be possessed while he was still conscious. Cartesian dualism tends to privilege the mind over the body, but in Gao's predicament, the bodily loss of control presented a moment of a new interiorized subjectivity.

I checked with Gao's wife, a robust woman in her early fifties. She told me that she did not believe her husband was mentally ill, just a little bit "deviated" (*pianle*). She asked me what I thought about the therapeutic treatment, and I found myself at a loss to advocate immediately the psychotropic foundation of cure. I asked if she had sought other means of help. Her no-nonsense reply was "these masters are just magicians. Sometimes they can help, but mostly they just perform. I know my husband is not mentally ill, but where else can I go?" The families of qigong patients were no different from families of other mentally ill patients. Faced with demands on financial and emotional resources, as well as the legal responsibility of taking care of their own, they managed to overcome quite difficult challenges.

Qigong narratives were compelling because they revealed the startling disjuncture between traditional health practice and the total therapeutic order to which these patients were eventually submitted by family members. Unsupervised encounters with qigong unleashed intense emotional experiences that challenged individuals. While healers had mastered these moments and could move beyond to harmonizing chaotic elements, novices who could not handle the power unleashed through qigong practices were unable to maintain a steady path. Rather than finding order and relief from qigong healers, these individuals instead faced existence inside the psychiatric hospital.

CULTURE-BOUND OR PRACTICE-SPECIFIC?

Does qigong deviation exist outside China? Rather than thinking of it as a culture-bound disorder solely tied to a specific culture, it may be necessary to think of qigong deviation as linked to the cultures of qigong practice that in the past decade have become transnational. In the fall of 1993, I received an anonymous call from an American who was the friend of a German practitioner. Calling from Arizona, she described the symptoms of what sounded like a serious case of deviation. Her friend had a history of depression and had taken up qigong to alleviate chronic symptoms of headache and malaise. Soon afterward, he began to talk nonstop, claiming to feel superhuman, and did not sleep for several nights. I quickly urged the caller to seek medical advice and the help of any qigong masters or martial arts teachers for her friend in Germany as soon as possible. The call for help indicated to me that qigong deviation was not just culture specific but could also be practice specific. In comparative interviews in California, practitioners have indicated varying degrees of mild deviation that were alleviated with the help of masters or simply by discontinuing all practice. According to Lim and Lin (1996), a Chinese American patient was treated for schizophreniform disorder brought on by qigong-reactive psychosis. After taking up qigong practice to treat his problems with kidney stones, the patient began to hear voices and believed he could communicate with aliens. After seeking the help of qigong masters, his wife ultimately contacted a psychiatrist, who provided antipsychotic medication. In the diverse and wildly unregulated world of martial arts outside China, laypeople mention otherworldly experiences that can occur either during or after practice. In *Martial Arts Madness*, Glenn Morris (1998) presents practitioner stories of "being attacked," visited by animals, or having other visions following meditation. Symptoms similar to qigong deviation have been noted by organizations that aid in the recovery of former cult members. In 2001, a BBC correspondent reported that a British qigong master who opened her own school claimed that conversations with Jesus and the twelve disciples enhanced her healing abilities.[4]

THE STATE AS CARETAKER

In comparing the overlapping categories of zhouhuo rumo and qigong psychosis, it was clear that masters believed that qigong psychosis was a preventable and manageable condition, such that a practitioner could even continue cultivation after developing symptoms. When patients were brought to TCM clinics, they were likely to receive a combination of acupuncture, herbs, and drug therapy. In the eyes of medical doctors, however, qigong deviation overlapped too much with mental illness. Rather than treating the disorder with traditional medicine, psychiatrists developed treatment based on biomedical modalities of drug therapy, rest cure, and cessation of practice. Both masters and many TCM practitioners had a ready cure, yet why did qigong deviation become privileged as a psychiatric category? Pathologization, as Foucault has argued, has the profound power to shape subjectivities and to centralize institutional authority. Though culture-bound syndromes may seem to be the most appropriate way to categorize the symptoms found in zhouhuo rumo, such classifications are not without inherent cultural values and political meaning.

The narratives of qigong deviation I heard indicated a strong need for careful management of qigong practice on the part of practitioners and teachers. Many individuals sought qigong primarily as a response to chronic illness and disorders with little understanding of the pathological conditions that could be exacerbated or instigated by improper practice. The growing number of clinical cases in 1990 came to be cited as justification for state regulation of qigong masters and practice. The occurrence of qigong deviation in contemporary urban China revealed how mystical experience challenged the very foundations of scientific order that the socialist bureaucracy sought to promote. The recent position of the Chinese socialist bureaucracy toward qigong associations and masters indicates great concern about the revitalistic and political potential of such formations. Although qigong continues to be promoted by the state as a unique Chinese tradition, the social networks of charismatic leaders represent a latent danger. Popular associations resonate with a long tradition of millenarian movements and peasant uprisings. Despite possible manifestations of disorder on both an individual and a social level, qigong remained quite popular.

CHAPTER FIVE

CHINESE PSYCHIATRY AND THE SEARCH FOR ORDER

STREET ENCOUNTERS with *fengzi* (mad people) in post-Mao China were occasionally described to me by acquaintances or friends with mixed feelings of pity and fear. More often, however, these figures were simply ignored. In my initial years in China as an English teacher, I often walked by the busy evening market on campus.[1] During the mid-1980s most state-owned vendors offered produce and goods at set prices. Grain, oil, and steamed bread were still rationed, however, so one needed special coupons to purchase these items. At 5:00 P.M., huge flats of steaming fresh tofu would arrive. Teachers, administrators, and commuters on their way home wound their way through the bustling and crowded path, pushing bikes with newly bought produce or fish in string bags on the handlebars. To the side of the main vendors, rural peddlers briskly sold fruits unavailable in stores. Other "free market" entrepreneurs (*getihu*) included self-employed workers who opened small bike repair stands or shoe repair stops on street corners. The familiar market scene altered dramatically for me in the fall of 1985 when a young woman in her thirties appeared out of nowhere and began marching in the middle of the market while fervently shouting decades-old slogans. I looked around, wondering what would happen next. Instead of a huge crowd forming to stare, most people appeared indifferent. Vendors and customers continued their transactions, only moving out of the way if she bumped into them. Her loud shouts were lost in the cacophonous swell of street hawkers' cries and bicycle bells. I turned to a nearby vendor to ask who the woman was and why no one seemed to care. He shook his head, stating that he wasn't sure but thought maybe she was mentally ill.

In the months after this incident, I would occasionally spot the same woman on other parts of campus, quietly walking and no longer shouting political slogans. Eventually, from students and colleagues, pieces of her story came together. Xiao Ma was the daughter of a university teacher who had been harshly criticized during the Cultural Revolution. Since that time, she would occasionally wander the streets, especially the market, and break into strident marches or songs. Her story and other riveting narratives of family separation, political denouncement, and dislocation that I encountered during my first two years in China led me to examine how mental health was constructed and practiced in post-Mao China. I was motivated by questions such as, How were people's lives affected by the profound political and economic transformations that constitute most of twentieth-century Chinese history? How does one frame an understanding of mental illness and mental health that encompasses these social changes? On my return for field research, I occasionally noticed other figures who appeared to be mad. At a major thoroughfare behind Qianmen, an older man dressed in rags waved a fan gracefully while executing dance steps, oblivious to the rush of bicycles, motorcycles, and cars weaving around him. No one seemed to glance at him as they jostled for space during the late afternoon commute home. On signposts or in local dailies, small black-and-white photos were posted with accompanying descriptions of mentally ill relatives missing from home.

Madness in twentieth-century Chinese literature and film tends to be represented by an iconic figure who moves from being rational but unthinking into a mental breakdown that allows him or her to see the "reality" of untenable social and political conditions (Lu 1990). The clarity of vision and fearlessness that come with madness in Chinese fictional accounts is very close to Shakespearean madmen such as Hamlet and King Lear who spoke the "truth." Despite the ubiquity of mad people in fiction, there was very little discussion in literature or media about the struggles that afflicted individuals and their families suffer in their daily lives. My interest in mental health was in one sense a response to the profoundly emotional narratives that I heard from students, colleagues, friends, and even strangers. What might be productive ways to understand psychiatry both as an institution with multiple pasts and as a new entity in the making? In seeking answers to all these questions, I decided to conduct ethnographic research in Chinese psychiatric clinics and hospital wards.

For Xiao Ma, the "ten years of chaos" (*shinian dongluan*), a euphemism for the Cultural Revolution, were enough for students, colleagues, and friends to explain her bouts of madness. In seeking the social interpretations of her behavior, I soon learned that such notions were quite elastic depending on the context and content. The ephemeral nature of madness and social constructs of normality were also poignantly highlighted for me when I spoke to patients and their family members in the asylum. Their stories reflect a broader concern about the formation of categories and the messiness of events that led to state-induced order. While medical accounts of culture-bound syndromes tend to be framed with an unwavering scientific gaze on categorical behaviors, sanitized of the messiness of clinical encounters, the lived experiences of individuals with these behaviors are anything but routine. For the many people involved at every point of the diagnosis and treatment, especially for patients, family members, neighbors, colleagues, doctors, and nurses, there is an emotional search for a cure to the sufferer's woes and the attainment of normality.

This chapter weaves together ethnographic accounts about the institutionalization of madness with historic accounts about the development of social order in twentieth-century China. My main intention is to show how psychiatry is an intersection between practice and ideology. Moreover, Chinese psychiatry has multiple layers of history and practice over different generations of doctors and diagnostic categories. The mundane everyday drama of caring for a family member acting out of order when one's own resources are depleted has rarely been addressed. For an anthropologist of psychiatry, discovering how certain norms become deeply embedded and unquestioned is as important as examining categories of strange or deviant behaviors. Medicine is a powerful window on humanity and social times. In the social sciences, health care is often gauged as an indicator of the overall health of a body politic. Writers such as Lu Xun and Chekhov, who were trained in medicine, turned to literature as a vehicle for their social vision. Lu Xun (1990), a celebrated author of the 1930s and once a medical student in Japan, wrote passionately about the clash of belief systems and the promise of modern life in his short story "Medicine." Psychiatry offers an additional lens through which to view the complex relations and tenuous boundaries among self, other, and society. Because the profession simultaneously deals with the mind and social categories of behavior, anthropologists have engaged with institutional ideologies and practices as ethnographic sites.

My research in Chinese mental hospitals was based on such anthropological studies of psychiatry with emphasis on the relation between official practices and alternative forms of mental health care. While questioning the modes of treatment, beleaguered parents, spouses, and children also remarked on how social norms had changed. The pursuit of personal leisure activities and alternative healing would not have been possible in the Maoist era. China's embrace of global capitalism, which meant an opening to international market forces abroad and the adoption of market economics at home, gained momentum during the 1980s and then again in the 1990s. Such changes over a relatively short period have led to a vast number of self-help publications as well as media coverage.

In the first half of this chapter, I provide an ethnographic orientation to everyday activities and routines in the psychiatric ward. I then outline the historic and institutional foundations of psychiatry in China. Tracing the transformations of Chinese psychiatry to particular moments of translation reveals how much this profession and its institutions are integral to national platforms for mental health and desires for social order. In linking the formations of psychiatry in China with the influence of foreign institutions and practices, it is important to keep in mind that there are "multiple histories of psychiatry" and institutional structures (Micale and Porter 1994). Western psychiatry itself has never been homogeneous or uniform. There have been significant differences in philosophies and forms of confinement across Europe, the United States, and the former Soviet Union.

IN A CHINESE ASYLUM

The term "asylum" (*bingfang*) is used for institutions that deal with ill patients, especially mentally ill. As a much-needed social space, like the public park, the asylum was one of the few official places in China where suffering could be expressed. As the arena where families could begin to restore a fragile sense of order in their lives, the hospital was also simultaneously the center from which the state developed an agenda of social order. The order prescribed by the state depended on the psychiatric hospital as the provider of mental health care. Such centers only occupied the peripheries of the larger stage that the Chinese socialist state was actively constructing for the Asian Games in 1990.

During my field research from 1990 to 1991, I visited three large metropolitan psychiatric hospitals, one provincial mental hospital, an industrial outpatient clinic, and a county psychiatric ward. The majority of my discussion will relate to the metropolitan centers where most of my fieldwork took place.

In the winter of 1990, after the Spring Festival (Chinese New Year) celebrations, the streets became silent with snow. In contrast to the gray hush outdoors, the hallways of the Institute of Mental Health were filled with cheerful noise. Convivial laughter between patients and staff members was quite a common occurrence. There was also a great deal of physical contact between patients, reminiscent of other social settings such as college dorms or factories.

My arrival required that I be given an appropriate identity. The vice director of the hospital, who had worked at the institute for over three decades, was in charge of my clinical studies. After showing me what would serve as my desk and locker on the third floor, I was given a white lab coat with a number on its pocket. Vice Director Chen then took me for a tour of the hospital. To an outsider, the clinics seemed like the setting for a drama. My initial impression of the outpatient waiting room was one of chaos. Cleaners were constantly mopping, and thus the floors reeked of disinfectant. There was constant movement, with doors forever opening and closing. As most patients were accompanied by at least one or two people, the crowd in the waiting room spilled into the hallways, where everyone had to dodge the ever-moving mop of the hospital cleaners. Similar to other hospitals throughout China, all doctors, including the director, vice director, senior doctors, and researchers, shared outpatient clinic duties in weekly rotation. Besides the general psychiatric clinics, there were also special clinics that focused on psychotherapy, neuropsychiatry, and even male impotency.

A visitor's first sight of the psychiatry hospital was the gate with a small sign in white and black letters. A clerk sitting in a little office next to the entrance served as the gatekeeper. Family members lined up at the clinic gate by seven in the morning. Some came by bus from outlying districts two hours away. City residents might bicycle twenty to thirty minutes to reach the clinic. Relatives first registered and paid fees. There were different scales depending on whether fees were paid by the work unit (*bao xiao*) or the individual (*zi fei*). After registering, one received a ticket and began the interminable waiting with other families and patients. By 8:00 A.M., everyone was huddled in the waiting room and cavernous hallways echoing with sounds of shuffling feet, closing doors, nurses calling numbers, and the eternal swishing of the hospital worker mopping the floors with murky water. Before entering the even smaller clinical offices, which were shared by several psychiatrists, many family members had already waited for an hour or more to get registered. Finally, the relatives and patients were called into the examination room to see the doctor. If the patient was new, a medical history had to be taken, about a twenty-five-minute process. If the patient was a regular, the doctor usually talked to the family members first (for an average of ten minutes) and then saw the patient (for less than five minutes). Doctors normally saw ten patients during each of their morning and afternoon shifts.

Despite the crowded clinical conditions and frenetic activity, it was inside the clinics that a space was created where a full range of emotions could be exhibited freely and without hesitation by family members and patients alike. My preconceived notions of privacy and personal space were challenged in this setting. Sometimes two consultations would take place in the same room, complete with accompanying relatives and other staff. A small eight-by-ten-foot

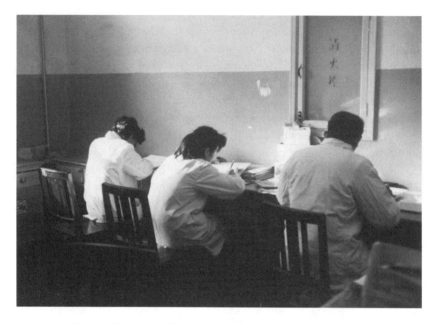

12. Resident psychiatrists updating medical histories

room could have up to ten persons squeezed inside, all talking loudly. Constant disruptions, such as the admission nurse peeking in or lost relatives looking for the room where their appointment was to take place, made it nearly impossible for a patient ever to be alone with a physician.

In the inpatient wards, the nurses' station consisted of a small room with two tables facing each other and wooden benches. Here nurses updated information in patient records or consulted doctors' instructions for specific patients. The station was open to any staff; inpatients, however, were kept out by a large locked door with a small opening at shoulder height. The resident psychiatrists, approximately eight to ten doctors in their twenties or thirties, were all frantically writing up cases at their desks in a small anteroom next to the nurses' station (see fig. 12). The resident psychiatrists often commented that every minute of interaction with patients or family members generated several pages in the histories. Most psychiatrists spent hours each day writing up daily entries. The medical histories became the official record of a patient's experience within the ward. While patients kept personal journals to record their progress for staff members, little of these narratives was included in the history. Instead, the daily records kept by nurses and the entries by psychiatrists became the primary source of knowledge about the patient. Interviews with fam-

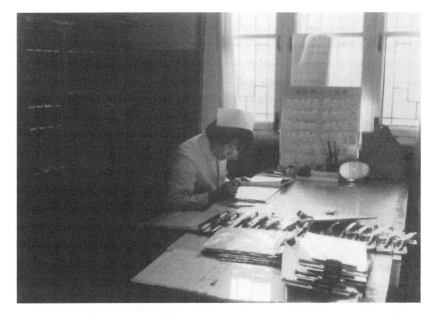

13. Nurse updating information on patients

ily members and outpatient clinical entries would also be included. The records room where all medical histories were kept was outside the clinic near the gated entrance. Its prominent place yet near invisibility to the rest of the hospital reflected the monumental but unseen labor that both doctors and nurses undertook (see fig. 13).

In contrast to North American hospitals, where the entryway is the key site of security, with staff windows, electronic locks, or buzzers, I found the entrance to the inpatient ward secured with only a simple deadbolt lock. There were three main inpatient wards: male, female, and cadres/foreigners wards. Each ward was located on a different floor and connected by an internal stairwell that was only open during afternoon activity hours and family visiting days. I was given a key to the wards after a few months. Originally, the administrators thought it would be simple enough for me to knock each time I wished to enter; however, this procedure soon became a nuisance to the physicians and staff in the wards, and so I was given a key.

All patients were assigned hospital pajamas (hierarchy was visible in the dress code: patients wore striped pajamas, female nurses wore small pointy hats, and doctors wore white coats) and then given lockers in which to stow their belongings—usually food items or books. No timepieces or jewelry were allowed.

Their daily lives were intensely scheduled from 5:30 A.M. to 10:00 P.M. each day. Alliances of patients within the wards did not always go according to diagnostic categories. Most friendships and conversations took place in the sleeping quarters after meals or during recreation periods when patients could walk after their slumber. Initially, most new patients would be quite reluctant to discuss openly the reasons they were there. New admittees were the objects of careful scrutiny not only by the hospital staff but also by other patients. Staff members responded to the patients routinely, according to the diagnosis; however, the patients tended to retain popular stereotypes of insanity and apply them to each other. Within the wards, there was a hierarchy among patients depending on their diagnostic category. Patients diagnosed with depression or admitted for psychosomatic disorders such as neurasthenia or obsessive-compulsion were unwilling to associate with chronic schizophrenics or bipolar manic-depressive patients. The tendency of patients was to focus on the content, origin, and social relations of illness rather than its formal classification. Family members were more anxious about the management of illness, hence frequent consultations with doctors took place.

Inside the wards, patients frequently milled around aimlessly from meal to meal. As a new person in a white coat coming into their lives, I was the focus of intense inquiry. The patients in the women's ward assembled around me—I was reminded of the first day of junior high school—and bombarded me with questions in Mandarin.

"What is your name, doctor? Who are you here to see?"

"I'm not a physician. I'm a researcher here to study mental health care in China."

"Are you Chinese?" the chorus asked.

"I'm Chinese American."

"Oh, I can speak English," chimed a university student.

The chorus continued, "Where are your parents?"

"They are in America. I was raised there."

The information was transmitted from the small circle around me to the other inpatients at large.

"What do your parents do?"

"How much money do they make?"

Knowledge is power. But even in a white coat, I was uncomfortable with the mantle bestowed on me and the identity created by the questions that were raised. I realized that what seemed highly personal questions were the standard queries put to any stranger in a new setting. In another sense, the questions mimicked the battery of questions in a psychiatric interview. But the tables were turned: rather than the patients being interrogated by authority figures in white coats, I was the one being poked and prodded by questions. It was certainly an informative experience, a role reversal that made me pay more attention later when I asked for personal information. Before I had time to continue addressing the growing circle around me, the vice director intervened to let me know it was lunchtime, breaking up the crowd and saying, "They are all curious about you." I later found out that there had been a general discussion of my background during a hospital staff meeting before I arrived. However, like a patient, I only pieced this together gradually as nurses or physicians would make reference to their preconceptions about me.

The case history, in which the medical history of a patient was discussed in detail, was both a pedagogical tool and a ritual. Once a week, each ward held team meetings of all physicians and nurses, led by the head psychiatrist, to discuss patient progress. A circle of staff members numbering about eighteen to twenty people all crammed into a tiny room and sat on wooden benches to attend the dramaturgy of that week's patient oration and questioning by the team. The meeting began with a recitation of patient history by the attending doctor. The patient was then brought in to be questioned about his or her case. Immediately afterward, the ritualized process of discussion began. I was introduced as a visiting Ph.D. research student and sat around the table with the other doctors. I soon realized that I would have to learn the language of Chinese psychiatry, which was entirely absent from my colloquial Mandarin. A whole new lexicon and world of classifications unrolled before me during these sessions, as doctors debated diagnoses and nurses raised questions about appropriate medication. It was during these group discussions and reflections on individual cases that I gained enough experience to acquire an intuitive sense of what constituted a particular category of mental illness.[2]

Once patients were committed for inpatient care, family members no longer had contact with them until the official visiting hours on Thursday and Sunday afternoons. These days were greatly anticipated by patients whose family members visited regularly. For those whose families lived far away and could not commute regularly, the time was spent quietly in the wards alone. Patients without visitors were not allowed to go to the activity hall because there was already so little room for families and staff members. Staff members would call out the names of patients as their family members came to call. During these days, I would alternate between spending time with patients who stayed in the ward and taking time to meet visiting family members. Each patient was allowed only two visitors at a time because of space limitations. Guests had to register at the front gate; then, at the main entrance to the locked courtyard where the patients waited, they would receive a wooden tag with the name of the patient they were visiting. Once inside the courtyard, the visitors would

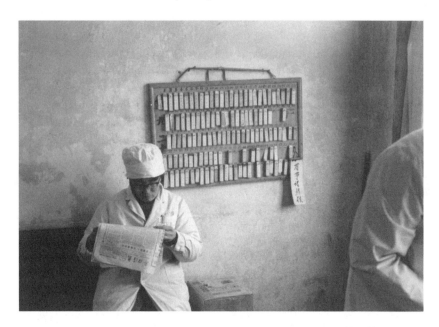

14. Wooden tags with the names of inpatients are given to visitors before they enter the grounds

wait until the name of the patient they were visiting was called out (see fig. 14). If weather permitted, families and patients would remain outside for the duration of the visit; if not, they would crowd into the activity room.

The recreational room during visiting hours was packed with people sitting in all possible areas, camped out with fruit and other food not offered by the standard hospital diet (see fig. 15). The scene resembled the waiting area in a train station, but the atmosphere hummed with intense activity and conversation. Parents peeled fruit for their children; adult children came to visit elderly parents with care packages; spouses would brought their children to see their partners in the clinic. But the main activity took place in the corners and stairways, where hospital residents and nurses were surrounded by family members asking about their patient's progress and the prognosis for the coming week. Everyone kept whispering questions about the patient's drug regimen, diet, and sleep patterns, along with the eternal query "How much longer?" These images of families remain with me: I saw and felt the concern and shared trauma of living with mental illness and the search for ways to counter the disruptions that had occurred in all these lives.

Whether the patient was a child, parent, or spouse, family members were deeply involved in the diagnosis, treatment, and sometimes even patient care

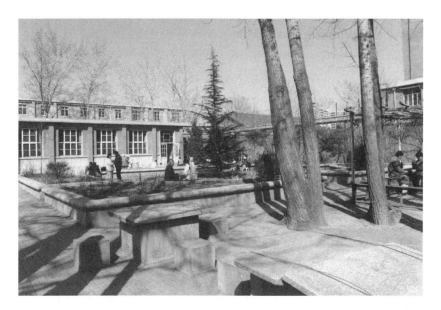

15. A quiet moment together during visiting hours

(depending on family finances). Some relatives would go to extensive efforts to visit, such as sitting on hard seats for train rides of several nights in order to seek better mental health care in Beijing. Most families brought food and personal items such as books and magazines, soap and toiletries, or letters and photographs. Each family would immediately huddle together, and the visitors would shower the patient with favorite foods or presents. "I always make these dumplings for my daughter; she doesn't like the food in here," one concerned mother told me after I greeted her. A male patient bounced his young son on a knee as his wife relayed stories about relatives who could not visit. Other male patients stood outdoors and smoked with relatives. Some patients openly sobbed in the arms of their spouses, parents, or children, begging to go home and relating their experiences inside the ward.

During the first few family visiting days, I awkwardly stood by, feeling as if I were intruding on private moments. As I gradually got to meet each patient in the wards, during later family visits the relatives would greet me and include me in their intimate circles. "We hear you are an American," said one patient's parents. "But you look just like us. Have a piece of fruit." Eventually, I looked forward to the visits as much as the patients. The visiting hours were also an opportunity for staff members to meet with relatives. During the brief consultations, psychiatrists gave updates on responses to medication and observed the behavior of the patients. Some patients were given a diagnosis on admittance, while a few cases were placed on hold until further observation. If the diagnosis was undetermined, families engaged in anxious conferrals with doctors during visits. I was constantly approached by relatives who presumed that I was a doctor. Family members and patients were all concerned with finding the appropriate category and were not relieved until a label had been established.

Departures were always difficult. Fruit peelings and sunflower seed shells lay scattered on tables and floors. The nurses would make a general announcement that visiting hours were over and went to each gathering to remind visitors to clean up. As the patients slowly ambled back into the wards, an attendant would check each parcel to make sure the contents were acceptable. Food items were acceptable, but cigarettes were confiscated to be rationed later. Patients were expected to eat dinner afterward, but often many were too full or sad to eat. The visits reminded patients of the lives they still had outside of the mental hospital.

The illness experience was not simply borne by patients; rather, it was a continuum of relationships managed and constantly negotiated in relation to state institutions. Whether acute or chronic, the burden of mental health care rested squarely on the shoulders of family members. Family units and the intricate network of social relations within this web of kinship had to reconstitute themselves in the face of tremendous changes, especially over the latter half of the twentieth century. The disruptions of political upheavals, separations, and generational differences have immensely affected the lives and experiences of all families in China, as is documented so well by the Kleinmans' work (1996, 1994) and in the volume by Davis and Harrell (1993). The relations and narratives of Chinese families in the late twentieth century reveal the flexible and reflexive character of these social and moral worlds.

THE WOMEN'S WARD

Conducting research in inpatient wards differed greatly from doing so in the outpatient clinics. In the outpatient setting, my role was limited to observations and occasional questions because of the large numbers of patients and family members waiting to be seen. The doctor in charge faced the formidable task of juggling care for new visitors and old patients; this sometimes involved ten to twelve consultations per morning or afternoon session. I did my best to fit into the scene without getting in the way. By contrast, the inpatient ward seemed like an oasis of calm. It was easier to conduct longer interviews in the women's ward (see fig. 16).

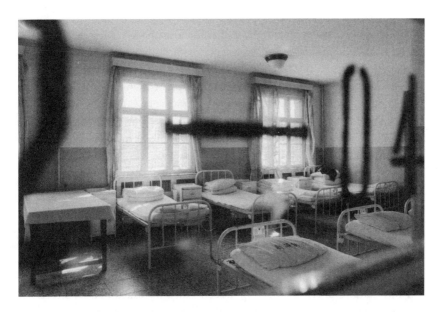

16. A group room in the women's ward

The Chinese hospital occupies a particular space in contemporary society and post-Mao literature. In her essay "Women, Illness, and Hospitalization," writer Zhu Hong (1994) argues that hospitals are an emblem of the social system itself. The Chinese madwoman in the popular realm drowns herself or otherwise commits suicide because of lost love, is a suffering mother, wanders the streets shouting, or ceases to speak. These images of madness stigmatize the experiences of women patients. Engendered psychiatry affects not only the specific experiences of female patients but, more important, the forms of classification management and discipline that take place in the psychiatric realm.

The field of mental health and practices of psychiatry have profoundly shaped the experiences of women and their bodies in every context of the profession. In the hospitals where I worked, women were not only patients but also caregivers such as nurses, psychiatrists, and administrators. My discussion here will address ways in which gender and psychiatry intersect. During the nineteenth century, naturalizing discourses of pathology determined that female bodies that did not fulfill social expectations of reproduction were hysteric (Martin 1987). In addition, classifications of mental illness such as psychosomatic disorders and depression were primarily used in the diagnosis and eventual uneven institutionalization of women in the West. In the twentieth century, certain categories and patterns of medication were specifically linked to women's mental disorders.

Some areas of contemporary psychiatry have been increasingly associated with gender. An incident that illustrates this took place on a hot summer day in July 1990 when I was interviewing Ms. Zhang, a woman in her forties, in Shandong Province. When asked why she was brought to the county asylum, her reply was, "It's no surprise I'm here. I'm at war [da zhang] with my family. I opened a sapphire mine last year, and the mine was quite prosperous. My husband and his relatives thought I should turn the money over to them, and I refused. This is my money that I've earned with bitter sweat and tears. No one believed that I would be able to find anything in there, and no one helped me. I started out by myself at first and then gradually hired people to help me. Now I have five workers in there. I pay them a monthly salary and a bonus."

I was quite surprised by this response and then remarked that it seemed her dispute might be settled more appropriately through the court system rather than a psychiatric system. To this Zhang replied, "I howled with anger [when they confronted her] and told them [her in-laws] that they would have to kill me before I gave up my livelihood. So they tied me up and brought me here. This is the only place I can't escape or get back at them." The attending psychiatrist corroborated Ms. Zhang's story of being a self-made woman who had serious family disputes. However, he also said the hospital was an important place that could provide rest and distance for all concerned.

As is the case in psychiatric institutions in the United States and elsewhere, patients can be admitted for observation, evaluation, and treatment for periods of several days to months. In urban China, the standard inpatient stay was two months (compared to two weeks in the United States). In rural areas, families and individuals shoulder the burden of hospital fees. Ms. Zhang was under evaluation for one week and was treated for hysteria (with sedatives) and eventually released. She was most unusual in being the owner of a mine. More specifically, her role and labor outside the home were being contested by in-laws, who viewed the proceeds of her efforts as belonging to them. In doctor interviews, family members talked about her uncooperativeness, irritability, and madness expressed in violence. Her refusal to respect standard gender roles and acknowledge traditional expectations was considered a form of deviant behavior.

Another interview, in the urban metropolis of Shanghai, indicated the increasing concerns young women face in an expanding market economy, such as adjusting to new values and body images. Xiao Dou, a slender young inpatient aged sixteen, talked to me about her desire to go home. When I asked why she was there, her reply was, "I don't like to eat all the time. My parents and grand-parents are always giving me food, and I'm trying to lose weight. . . . The doctors here tell me I have a disorder similar to Karen Carpenter who died of not eating. I know now that my problem might be similar, but I'm not like her at all." Needless to say, I was surprised to find this young girl already an inpatient in the mental ward. I asked the doctors and nurses why they had decided to admit her. Nurse Wang replied, "We need to restore the vitality of the young girl's desire to eat and be a part of her family again." Dr. Zhou answered, "She, like many other young girls in China, is becoming concerned about her appearance, and this is quickly becoming an obsession. We are not using psychotherapeutic drugs as much as psychotherapy and IV feeding. She will be discharged once she has gained her original weight back." Xiao Dou remained in the hospital for three weeks, when she had regained some plumpness in her cheeks and showed more willingness to eat. Her mother and other family members showed their concern by visiting every day with offerings of food. Dr. Zhou mentioned that it was not unusual for some patients, especially those diagnosed with eating disorders, to return again.

Newly emerging categories in Chinese psychiatry, such as eating disorders, could be said to accompany different patterns of consumption and materialism. These new categories are not only historically specific but also linked to global notions of women's bodies and their functions in society. The two cases I have briefly discussed both stood out for me as situations where gender roles shared a particular intersection with psychiatric management. In the post-Mao period of decollectivization and increased consumption, psychiatric classifications incorporated global standards of practice and categories.

One day in August, after I had returned from a visit to the county rural psychiatric hospital, one of the inpatient residents, Ms. Feng, took me aside in the women's ward. She was an engaging woman of slight build in her thirties. Even after a six-week stay in the hospital for neurasthenia, she had not gained weight like the other patients. Mrs. Feng presented me with a chart. "It includes all the information you need for your study. While you were away, we inpatients discussed your project. We worried that your study would be incomplete without our help, so we decided to help you finish. Look, here is Mrs. Wang's information. She wanted to be included before she left last week." On the chart were carefully tabulated rows of data: names, ages, educational statuses, occupations, diagnoses, and medication histories. I was speechless and touched. When I looked up, a handful of the women patients who were also sitting in the dorm room stood around admiring the elaborate chart I had been presented. The collective effort represented not only concern for exact statistics but also the care with which they observed my behavior and their hopes to be involved in their representations. Like the elaborate handwritten medical histories patients presented in clinical consultations, these women felt compelled to present their own classifications to me as an anthropologist.

My encounters in the women's ward made me reflect on the ways in which psychiatric care had been organized in the past. In what follows, I explore the historical strands that contribute to the current moment of practice.

FROM MADNESS TO MENTAL HYGIENE

Understanding the story of psychiatry in China entails tracing evolving cultural categories of normality as well as contextualizing the selective engagement with theories and practice, professionalization, and global diagnostic standards. In following the development of psychiatry, certain narratives of modernization and professionalization are intricately linked to the historic contexts of political and social transformations. Madness as a social category continues to be a wellspring of public imagination in China. In contemporary Chinese literary and film contexts, madness has usually been portrayed as an inevitable response to unbearable social and political circumstances in both feudal as well as modern times. The social chaos of political movements in China and the search for order by various regimes have been recurrent themes in the twentieth century. Lu Xun's well-known *Diary of a Madman* (*Kangren Riji*), written in the 1920s, tells the story of one person who grows increasingly suspicious of others and eventually resorts to eating human flesh, the ultimate sign of insanity. While the central character might inspire horror in others, he is just as repulsed by the general public's inhumanity. The novel has been viewed by many as a social commentary and moral tale about a larger structure of social chaos that could only generate madness, with the individual experience of madness reflecting the wider context of social insanity. Even popular beliefs about madness continue to rely on dramatic images such as a mad person dancing in the street or an individual overcome by traumatic events that have fatal consequences.

Madness was recognized early in Chinese folklore and traditional medical writings and commonly associated with illness introduced into the body by winds. Shamanic healing by Daoist healers involved a wide range of treatments. Depending on the individual nature of the suffering, these prescriptions included ingesting the ashes of spiritual inscriptions, physical exercises, or forms of exorcism. Several key texts form the basis for medical classification and intervention. In the *Huangdi Neijing Suwen* (The Yellow Emperor's canon of internal medicine), a classic of state orthodox medicine, madness was differentiated into two main categories: *dian* (insanity) and *kuang* (violent, wild behavior) (Kao 1979; Ng 1990).

Though psychiatry did not exist as a specialization or institution in early imperial China, traditional medicine did address madness in terms of yin and yang imbalances. *Kuang*, where a person experienced an "uncontrollable desire to climb up high places, to chant, to sing, to disrobe in public, and to curse people," was attributed to excessive yang (Ng 1990, 33).[3] In contrast, *dian* was the condition where a person was very quiet, almost catatonic, and was associated with excessive yin. Most mental illnesses were associated with excessive emotions and the imbalance caused by such excess or deficiency in the internal organs of the body rather than solely located as mental disorders. Emotions were thought to have a powerful physical impact on the qi of a person, such as making qi rise, decline, leak, contract, or dissipate. During the Han period (206 B.C.–220 A.D.), physicians adhering to the *Shanghan lun* (Treatise on cold illnesses) considered susceptibility to cold and heat as cause for mental and physical instability. While herbal treatment and acupuncture were probably the most common therapies, during the late imperial period, experimental psychological therapies based on "emotional countertherapies" were also practiced (Sivin 1995, 2). Based on a systematic correspondence between the five elements and emotions such as anger, sorrow, grief, or fright, any imbalance could be counteracted with incidents that triggered the appropriate emotional response. During the Tang dynasty, winds that exacerbated *dian* or *kuang* were noted. "In the *Qianjin yaofang*, Sun finally established *feng* (wind) as a pathogenic agent for madness" (36). This association probably contributed to the term *fengzi* (mad person), which continues to be used in Chinese today to refer to the mentally ill.

Vivien Ng documents the shift of madness from mental illness to social deviance through Qing imperial court cases of insanity. Before the establishment of psychiatric clinics and before hospital beds were kept aside for psychiatric patients, most instances of insanity were kept within the domestic sphere. Even if the cases were attributed to spirit possession or environmental causes, family members were held responsible for any damages to property or social disruption. Consequently, most families tended to confine their mentally ill relatives at home, either tied to heavy furniture or locked up. Another strategy to avoid social stigma would be to abandon the mentally ill or allow them to wander away while in another town.[4]

During the late nineteenth century and early twentieth century, when most practice in China was conducted by Western missionary physicians, the emphasis on treatment often required extricating patients from families who refused to allow their relatives to be taken away to hospitals (Kao 1979). Most families still tried to keep the secret of mental illness tightly within the inner quarters of the home, hidden from the outside world. In the first decades after the establishment of the PRC, the fledgling mental health program began to introduce programs based on Soviet models of work therapy and Maoist forms of political engagement for psychiatric patients. Nonetheless, the social stigma of mental illness remained quite powerful and kept many families from seeking proper care for their relatives.

The alliance between state building and mental health in China has always been concerned with long-standing issues: providing for a large population and maintaining social order. The institution of psychiatry has had several ruptures in its organization and the social meanings of its practice. Such ruptures reflect ongoing political transformations and reveal some of the choices made in translating psychiatry within the Chinese context. As a form of specialized medicine that was introduced by missionary medical practitioners in the late nineteenth century, psychiatric institutions eventually became part of a larger program of national order and discipline in the first half of the twentieth century. During this century, the institution of psychiatry evolved, with the establishment of asylums, hospitals, teaching schools, journals, nursing associations, and other professional groups.

Rather than focusing solely on contemporary psychiatric terms and mental health categories, this chapter seeks to situate the practices of Chinese psychiatry within historical frameworks of cultural translation and national discourses of modernity. Terms, categories, and even spatial orders in psychiatry are inextricably linked to the contexts in which meanings and practices are adopted and utilized. Psychiatry in contemporary China is thus situated at particular intersections of cultural meanings of madness, international and national classification categories for mental illness, and evolving institutional practices.

Thinking about psychiatry in a cultural context offers opportunities to view the ways in which practices have been transformed by institutional discourses of modernity. Social histories of madness and cultural studies of institutions have been influenced by Foucault's writings on the history of madness and institutionalization (Rose and Miller 1986). While T. M. Luhrmann rightly points out that Foucault's focus on governmentality overshadows the suffering of individuals (2000, 11), Foucault's awareness of space that is radically transformed by mental illness is instructive. Foucault amplified the relationship between political practice and medical discourses in *The Birth of the Clinic* (1994) and *Madness and Civilization* (1973). In his essay "Politics and the Study of Discourse," he further remarks on these intersections: "What is transformed by political practice is not medical 'objects,' but the system which provides a possible object for medical discourse" (1994, 67). Institutionalization has been useful in placing bodies under a centralizing medical gaze, and Foucault's analysis of governmentality beginning at the corporeal level provides critical groundwork for understanding the rise of institutions.

Three historical contexts that mark the development of psychiatry have particular salience for the circulation of notions and forms of treatment in China: pre-1949 missionary, Maoist, and post-Mao global psychiatry. The use of the asylum and psychiatry in the treatment of mental disorders is quite distinct in each of these periods, and in each prevailing political discourse between global institutions and local conditions determined the uses of categories and forms of mental health care. "Modern" psychiatry, particularly what constitutes modern practice, continues to be revised and contested and can be viewed as a microcosm of social relations and power structures in conversation. Although mental illness was recognized early as a pathological state, the care of patients did not become a public concern until the late nineteenth century, when foreign medical missionaries began to organize support for public clinics. Despite the tremendous upheavals experienced from one governing body to the next, many socialist institutions of order, particularly psychiatry, had their beginnings in the early twentieth century rather than midcentury. But further psychiatric institutions in China were not built and did not become systematized until mental health became a massive state campaign under Mao in the 1950s. Significant differences between rural and urban health care are historically based.

MISSIONARY MEDICINE

Chinese psychiatry is embedded within missionary encounters of the late nineteenth century, when Western-trained physicians campaigned for more humane (i.e., Christian) treatment of the insane. The missionaries' implementation of psychiatry was part of their general concern for the mentality of Chinese people. The advocacy of Western medicine by Protestant missionaries further intensified during the late nineteenth century and especially during the Republican era of the 1920s and 1930s, as their clinics provided the only psychiatric services available to the general public. The fusion between Christian humanitarianism and American philanthropy merged with Chinese notions of modernism.

An 1849 report by Dr. Benjamin Hobson, who established the Hong Kong Missionary Hospital, mentions the relative infrequency of insanity in China: "Considering the phlegmatic temperament and temperate habits of the Chinese, it might be appreciated that this malady is not of frequent occurrence, and I think further inquiry will prove that insanity prevails to a much less extent in China than in Europe. . . . Lunatic Asylums are unknown in China" (Wang and Wu 1936, 361). The first psychiatric hospital, the Canton Refuge for the Insane, was opened in 1898 by Dr. Joseph Kerr, an American missionary who believed in clinical evangelism and occupational therapy for patients. Kerr was the designated heir to Dr. Peter Parker, who was the first Protestant missionary to establish a surgery practice in Canton. The establishment of the asylum took considerable effort and was a lifelong project for Dr. Kerr, who had a distinguished career, publishing several medical texts and developing teaching facilities in China.

Most medical missionaries emphasized surgery, particularly eye operations and removals of tumors; this drew an abundance of Chinese patients seeking immediate and visible results. Despite Dr. Kerr's considerable stature in the profession, there was marked reluctance from fellow missionaries and even more resistance from family members of potential patients. It wasn't until Kerr purchased three acres of his own land and sought assistance from private donors that the refuge was built; it opened just three years before his death. In contrast to the charity hospitals run by missionaries, the Kerr refuge was funded primarily by revenue generated from patient billing and donors. At the turn of the century, the bulk of patient referrals came from the local police and magistrates, who used the hospital as an overflow penal institution and paid the bills for housing patients, an early development of forensic psychiatry in China. The mental hospital remained open until 1927, when it closed in the face of continued controversy; a total of 6,599 cases had been admitted over the three decades it had operated (Wang and Wu 1936, 709). Later, some of the work was continued in other hospitals under the republican government. Until the establishment of the People's Republic in 1949, however, an assortment of private institutions and charities was the primary source of mental health care available in China. As the use of psychopharmacology was not yet integral to the treatment of patients, the treatment modalities of this time included rest cure, work therapy, and physical restraint for the worst cases. Small psychiatric wards as part of missionary hospitals eventually opened throughout Chinese provinces, but the profession was most firmly established in Canton.

Most of the missionary doctors had much difficulty convincing Chinese families to bring individuals into the hospital and even greater difficulty retaining patients, as many tried to run away. This was due in part to the social stigma of mental illness and also to the fear of being mistreated by foreigners, often referred to as foreign devils. Relatives preferred locking their mentally ill in attics or banishing them to the streets to allowing the "Other" or Western doctors to confine them. Dr. Kerr noted that the failure especially of the well-to-do and middle classes to adhere to new methods stemmed from general reluctance to seek help that would make public family secrets, such that few Chinese families made use of the asylum. Only when private offices were opened, where clients could pay for services anonymously, did more middle-class families come to the refuge. Later, after the turn of the century, members of the imperial family and other elite families contacted hospital administrators when the need arose. For instance, a memo by Dr. Andrew Woods to Dr. R. S. Greene, a Peking Union Medical College administrator, indicated a general's interest in seeking examination for his son as well as the son-in-law of a member of the imperial family.[5] Usually when such members were admitted, special wings or wards were opened up. (Such practices were in place at the hospital where I worked: the top floor was reserved for cadres (*ganbu*) and foreign visitors.) Western doctors also noted the need for separate units for foreigners who were in "a most difficult mental state" and "upsetting the entire ward."[6] Another, more desperately worded memo from Dr. Woods described the unavoidable admission of insane patients: "We now have two patients requiring guards; and last month we had three, all foreigners, who were mentally disturbed. The anxiety and strain involved in caring for such patients is considerable when facilities are but makeshift; and the opprobrium to be expected by the hospital will be uncomfortable to bear if we fail to care properly for them."[7]

In twentieth-century China, madness was mainly associated with haunting specters found on the street. Mad people who tore off their clothes and danced in the streets added to the chaos associated with urban spaces. The response involved local police, who were responsible for maintaining the streets as an arena of state order. In the 1920s Beijing rickshaw pullers and vagrants alike faced the wrath of the street police (Strand 1989). Disturbances of public order commonly ended with the street police bringing those responsible to the local jails. The alliance between the asylum and the police became even more explicit when local police and the Canton asylum came to a formal agreement at the turn of the century (Diamant 1993). Similar moves were taken by Beijing municipal police. By 1920 a year-end report entitled "PUMC and the Problem of Insanity in China" begins with an estimate of at least 10,000 mentally disturbed Chinese in Beijing.[8] The author continued with a call for the protection of the insane and prevention of their incarceration: "The institution in Peking which is called an asylum is really a prison for insane criminals." He also appealed for better education and training of physicians to deal with mental diseases. By 1933 transfer of the administration of the Municipal Insane Asylum from the Bureau of Social Welfare to the Health Department was completed.[9] Once under the aegis of Peking Union Medical College, specialized training for psychiatric doctors and nurses was part of the mission. The City

Psychopathic Hospital was unique for this special training of professionals. In 1933 a survey on neuropsychiatric beds in China revealed there were very few hospitals with special psychiatric wards or even beds.[10] At most, a general hospital might have a few beds for this purpose. There were very few hospitals with specially trained staff.

The work therapy model was quite a popular form of treatment in the missionary hospital context. Patients would produce small goods for several hours each day. Work was viewed as an antidote to mental instability and believed to promote moral character and hygiene. Such methods remain in use even today: most major institutions incorporate handicraft production as part of weekly therapy.

In sum, practices of psychiatry in the late nineteenth and early twentieth century were primarily carried out by Western missionary doctors with Chinese patients who were recruited from the streets or brought in by local authorities. Occasionally, Western-educated Chinese physicians were trained and practiced in the asylums. The psychiatric asylum was an important site at a time when notions of social order demanded the separation of madness from Chinese public spaces through the enforcement of police as well as the confinement of patients previously kept isolated in domestic spaces.

MENTAL HYGIENE AND SOCIALIST ORDER

Under socialism, mental health care was distinctive for its linkage of mental hygiene with public health. Public health during the 1950s was viewed as vital to the well-being of the nation. Campaigns against infectious diseases such as schistosomiasis and malaria along with sanitation projects in the "patriotic health movement" were undertaken (Sidel and Sidel 1973, 179). Mobilization of the nation and its new citizens coalesced in the development of generalists rather than specialists. New cadres of health care workers, the "barefoot doctors," offered primary health care to rural dwellers, making great strides in redressing historic patterns of inequality between rural and urban centers. Infant mortality decreased, while life expectancy rose. The emphasis on community-based care also spread to mental health care. Community beds were organized in collaboration with families; this made it unnecessary to build expensive hospitals. Mental health care at this time emphasized biological aspects of somatization rather than a psychosocial approach (Pearson 1995; Kleinman and Lin 1981).

The early socialist period, in the mid-twentieth century, was transformative with regard to official legislation for mental health and educational programs. In contrast to missionary psychiatry, where proponents worked closely with authorities to remove disruptive elements off the street, this new phase in Chinese psychiatry seemed to embrace mental health as a platform for developing the minds and hearts of the population. With the inception of the People's Republic of China, mental health care became intertwined with the idea of social progress. The first five-year plan (1958–1962) cited it as a top priority for a modernizing China focused on socialist revisions of policies and practices. But rather than continuing the institutions established by Western missionaries, a socialist model of mental hygiene (*jingshen weisheng*) embracing Soviet psychological theories and practice was established instead. Neologisms such as the asylum (*fengrenyuan*), psychiatric institution (*jingshenke bingfang*), mental hygiene (*jingshen weisheng*), and mental health (*jingshen jiankang*), in particular, are simultaneously embedded within Chinese social categories and professional definitions. The highly touted barefoot doctor program even included a segment on diagnosis and treatment of mental illness in the countryside. As new centers and hospitals were created, former missionary centers and practices were deemphasized.

Hygiene (*weisheng*) occupied particular prominence in Maoist campaigns for socialist transformations of mental illness, once viewed as a private burden, into mental disease that could be countered with work therapy and political reform. Mental hygiene (*jingshen weisheng*) was historically a term intended to counteract the social stigma and popular conceptions of mental illness. The category was thus part of larger public health initiatives that were linked to morality, in which both social and political forms of decay would be rehabilitated with socialist values and practice. The drive to get rid of decadence politicized many public health issues, especially mental health, as moral issues. Psychiatric institutions continue to be promoted as centers of medical science where mental illness can be treated as a disease and not as a social deviation. The image of psychiatry the state promotes is thus one of scientific objectivity in line with Marxist practice, a necessary part of the grand scheme for a "socialist civilization" (*shehuizhuyi wenming*) that Anagnost (1997) documents in her study of Chinese state discourse. Such a notion of mental health is also apparent in the term "mental hygiene" (*jingshen weisheng*), which is still used in reference to mental health care.

The Chinese use of Soviet models of mental health care in general practice did not entirely replicate its extreme "penal psychiatry," in which Soviet asylums were used to control and punish political dissidents.[11] Instead, new theories and modalities of treatment emphasized political engagement with socialist liberation models. The therapeutic system emphasized that the mentally ill could be retrained to become valuable citizens and model workers for a new society. In this vast social program of psychiatry for the people, there was a shift from the notion of the asylum as a way to confine madness to the use of psychiatric clinics and hospitals to rehabilitate the debilitating stigma of mental illness. In their study of Chinese psychology, Robert and Ai-ling Chen (1987) document the role of Soviet psychology in transforming notions of Chinese psychiatric practice during this period. Adherence to Pavlov's ideas led to the principle of "the development of certain abnormalities of mental function after exposure to overwhelming and exhausting stimuli, or to repetitive disturbing stimuli" (Wortis 1950, 136). Pathologized states, whether organic or social in origin, were still possible to reform and cure through activity and work; this was a central component of Pavlovian theory.

The political activism of the Great Leap Forward and the Cultural Revolution during the 1960s had immense impact on the practice of psychiatry. Again the emphasis was on work as an indicator of moral character and aptitude for socialist principles. While the factories attached to mental hospitals continued to produce socks, staplers, and screws, Pavlovian work therapy incorporated political activity; readings of Mao Zedong's writing were considered crucial to one's mental well-being. Such activities in socialist thought reform reflected larger social transformations outside the mental hospital, where all citizens were expected to read political works. To choose not to participate indicated one's reluctance to show reform and hence madness.

The ruptures in psychiatric practice were most dramatic during the Cultural Revolution (1966–76). Psychology was viewed as a decadent Western theory. The discipline of psychology was viewed as having a different intellectual genealogy in China, and the linkages to work therapy and the actual bodies of patients as subjects meant that psychiatry had a different political trajectory from the social sciences. The few clinics remained open, but some practitioners were expected to devote their time to political reeducation. A few psychiatrists managed to counsel secretly old patients and distraught family members who sought them in confidence. As one practitioner in his seventies recounted, "After the public performance of denouncing rightists, several families still continued to see me at night when they wouldn't be detected. I resorted to psychotherapy when I could not give them prescriptions." The perseverance of this psychiatrist and his patients shifted his later research in the post-Mao period to psychotherapy.

POST-MAO GLOBAL PSYCHIATRY

The post-Mao era of psychiatry has been distinct from previous eras for several patterns: increasing professionalization with uniform training, national conferences, NGO funding, international classification codes, and research publications. The development of the present-day profession is highly tied to

Ministry of Health allocations and international aid agencies, especially the World Health Organization. Like its Western counterparts, clinical psychiatry occupies a lower status in the medical profession compared to high-tech specialties such as neurosurgery. Like general hospitals, the main centers are located in the cities. There are eleven psychiatric research centers, including the Beijing Institute of Mental Health and the Shanghai Institute of Mental Health, the primary WHO model units. Status and organization are intricately linked to international funding. In the rural regions, mental health care is attached to local rural health care stations so that preventive and primary care can reach rural workers.

Health care in urban areas is vastly different from what is offered in the countryside. In rural areas, three tiers of health care are available. Most villages have part-time medical workers or rural doctors, once referred to as barefoot doctors. Such doctors are no longer barefoot and are no longer part of the commune or brigade system, both of which were disbanded under market reform. Many former barefoot doctors, however, remain members of their communities and work in rural enterprises. They are the primary source of health care and are trained to deal with simple illnesses, offer herbal medicine, or help in childbirth. In previous decades, these rural medics carried out public health programs in their communities. Rural township health centers provide the next level of service but tend to be less well equipped than county hospitals, the final level of health care in the countryside.

All Chinese cities and towns in the post-Mao era have hospitals, which increasingly offer more advanced medical technologies. In urban areas above the county level, there are specialized hospitals. These include military, industrial, collective-owned, joint venture, and state-owned hospitals. In addition there are also sanitariums, clinics, disease-prevention stations, maternity and child care centers, and privately operated medical facilities. In contrast to clinics with missionary origins, where psychiatric hospitals were private, mental health wards are now public and state owned. In 1948 there were only 1100 beds for 500 million people (a ratio of .22 bed per 10,000 people) with fifty to seventy trained physicians and even fewer nurses (Lin and Eisenberg 1985). By 1995 the number of beds significantly increased, to 120,000–130,000 beds, or about 1.1 beds per 10,000 people (Phillips, Pearson, and Wang 1994). By 2000 there were an estimated 77,000 mental health professionals ("Nation's Mentally Ill" 2000)

The number of beds is still quite low in comparison to what is available in other countries with smaller populations. For instance, even the largest city hospital in Beijing or Shanghai has only several hundred beds compared to self-contained psychiatric institutions in the West with 1000 to 5000 or more patients, minivillages that are self-sustaining. In keeping with recent trends in psychiatry, there is an increased usage of psychopharmacology in China. However, as K. M. Lin (1996) has shown, dosage levels for Chinese patients tend to be lower. Chinese psychiatry has been viewed with interest, particularly because it offers alternatives to Western psychiatric practices undergoing deinstitutionalization and managed care accounting.

Contemporary mental health care reflects larger social and economic transformations since the post-Mao reforms of the late 1970s. Like its counterparts in the rest of the world, Chinese psychiatry has been gradually integrating international diagnostic categories and psychotropic treatment with codes of Chinese classification since the 1980s. The development of mental health care began with an outreach by the post-Mao government to Western and overseas Chinese experts (Lin and Eisenberg 1985). Reforms in mental health care during this period sought to reverse the changes wrought by Maoist thought reform and psychiatric practices in the previous decades.

Mental health remains part of the public health structure framed within the language of development. In the present state of Chinese psychiatry, mental hygiene is intertwined with biomedical practices to underscore a prevailing state discourse on the need for order and normality. The Chinese asylum is the site of several intersecting forces and desires: transnational aid agencies and pharmaceutical corporations, embodiments of socialist modernization, and negotiations among family members. In an ironic twist of fate, this has involved a return to the very sites established by missionaries before 1949. A model rehabilitative center in the suburbs of Shanghai is based in the former physical structure of a French charity hospital. Grilled ironwork and gardens are only part of the physical and program restructuring taking place.

Today, early Western models of mental health care coexist with recently imported models of biomedicine, where scientific research and psychotropic drugs are increasingly emphasized in the treatment of mental patients. Political reforms introduced in the late 1970s and early 1980s allowed Chinese scholars and psychiatrists to participate in exchange programs abroad. By the time I started field research, the first wave of senior cadres had been visiting the United States and Europe for over a decade. The next generation of scholars went outside China during the 1980s at earlier stages of their careers to receive graduate degrees and postdoctoral training. International health organizations such as the WHO have opened collaborative centers for joint research and training. Along with the import of Western biotechnology, there was also the transfer of classification categories from the DSM-IV and ICD-10. Such use of screening tests is intended to align with global psychiatric practices.

The Chinese professional community is presently engaged in active translation of the latest Western psychiatric articles and international classification categories into Chinese. Such translations of categories in the Chinese Classification of Mental Disorders (CCDM-2R) are a critical exemplar of cultural translation. Despite all intentions to conform with international classification codes, the CCDM-2R includes specific additions, deletions, retentions, and variations, clear indicators that cultural meanings and differences are being negotiated (Lee 1996, 451). Urban centers are primarily in control of these translations, as the larger research hospitals and majority of professionals are located in cities.

In other regions, there is a slight time lag in the adoption of global psychiatric research. Even with the uniform use of the CCDM classifications in China, great regional differences remain, especially in hospital stays: during the early 1990s rural patients stayed an average of 37.2 days, and urban patients an average of 140, a gap attributable to work unit health care packages and insurance in urban regions. Most mentally ill inpatients are schizophrenic and tend to represent more severe cases because of the limited structure of diagnosis in rural regions. The diagnostic category of the patient greatly affects the forms of treatment from staff members and other patients. In larger psychiatric hospitals with over a hundred inpatients, 80 to 90 percent of the patient population consists of chronic schizophrenic patients for whom family care is no longer viable. The hospital in which I conducted fieldwork was primarily a research unit, and therefore there was a greater range of psychiatric disorders. While the majority of patients were still diagnosed as schizophrenic, there were also clinical cases of depression, neurological disorders, neurasthenia, and psychosomatic disorders.

In the process of updating psychiatric classification codes and practices to make them equivalent to international categories, mental hygiene (*jingshen weisheng*) is more often invoked to refer to programmatic or institutional approaches to mental health, while *jingshen jiankang* (mental health) is used when addressing individual cases. The discipline presently depends on institutional support and active dialogue among professional committees, state institutions, and international colleagues. Such engagements are crucial not only to localizing the global discourse of psychiatry but also to subject making. Post-Mao forms of professionalization in a sense unlinked mental health from public health by creating more alliances with psychology and basic research. Nonetheless, the Chinese psychiatric asylum functions as an official site of order and control for the disorderly and chaotic elements that emanate from within an individual rather than the social setting.

Rather than situating families in opposition to state institutions with regard to mental illness, most social welfare programs and psychiatric units rely on the family unit as an integral component of mental health care in China. The negotiations that family members engage in such as the ones outlined above are often directed by representatives of state units such as the hospital, work units, or public security. There is implicit recognition, however, that relatives are the primary caregivers, and outside the psychiatric ward, most families can seek a number of options. Inside the psychiatric wards, relatives try to be active in constructing possible options of diagnosis and treatment even as most have the least autonomy in directing the path of treatment of their inpatient relatives in this realm.

The involvement of family members in mental health care is often overlooked in discussions of the structure of psychiatry. Relatives of patients play significant roles in the maintenance of patients during their stays in the wards and even afterward. In spite of state expansion and a modernized mental health care system, the burden of mental illness stigma and responsibility remains with the family. As in Qing imperial times, family members are held responsible for patient care and costs, especially in chronic cases where an unemployed patient has no benefits. The steps that lead a person to be committed to the mental hospital are highly dependent on that individual's home situation and relations at work. Even if individuals are disruptive at home, most families do not bring them to the clinic until the family order is significantly disrupted. Many parents, spouses, and children are in tears speaking to the doctor of their family's distress and are still hesitant to have their relatives admitted. The social stigma of mental illness in China remains acute for afflicted individuals and their family members who seek mental health care despite interventions in the development of the asylum.

Many of the patients and their relatives whom I interviewed in ethnographic fieldwork cited the difficulty of sharing their distress with outsiders. To be open with neighbors or coworkers entailed the loss of face in social situations and even, in some cases, the loss of normal responsibilities at work. Seeking mental health care still involves a great risk and is always accompanied by the unspoken fear of being found out by one's neighbors or colleagues. Popular images of madness such as divine fools who dare to speak the truth or frenzied *fengzi* (mad persons) who run naked through the streets are often cited by Chinese as common examples of those with mental disorders. Such stereotypes resonate with popular images of lunatics of the past.

Although most inpatients did not wish to stay in the mental institution, their family members were more likely to comply with the hospital policy of a three-month stay. During interviews, family members stated that it was a good thing to have their relatives remain in the hospital as long as it took to cure them and also because the fragile order of family life could be somewhat restored in their absence. Most spoke of their reluctance to bring patients to the mental hospital yet felt they no longer had the emotional resources to withstand the constant disruptions and chaos that one individual had brought to their lives. The ninety-day period created a space in which order could be created. Mental health care, then, was viewed as an antidote to disorder in the household as well as in the individual. While the compliance of Chinese families with the therapeutic entity was thorough, it is important to emphasize that the family and work units were not collaborators with psychiatrists as evil agents of the state. Instead, the cultural fear of disorder and the ideal of harmonious relations were constantly at play such that mental health was promoted and viewed as an institution of order. The health care workers, family members, and work units were all involved in a genuine desire to help the patient because they wanted to maintain order and a sense of normality not only for the individual but also for the social body and body politic.

In recent years, family psychotherapy has become available, but only to a select few. This is due to the small number of therapists trained in this field as well as the general perception that patients need prescription drugs to be cured, not just the chance to talk about their family crises. Families may also seek advice and help outside the psychiatric unit through other avenues. One noteworthy trend has been hot lines that people may call for anonymous help. The Chinese popular press and magazines in recent years have published stories that deal with social issues such as madness. Besides seeking a range of clinical practitioners, whether TCM or biomedical, family members may write to newspapers or journals seeking advice and hope that a journalist will either investigate the situation or put them in contact with proper authorities. Official news organs such as *Renmin Ribao* (People's daily) or the *Jiankang Ribao* (Health daily) remain the primary means by which information about mental health care programs proliferate to the urban community.

In sum, there is an intimate relationship between contemporary state institutions and family involvement in the management of mental illness. This alliance is not always the smoothest as there is much contestation and negotiation not only between family and state but also among family members; however, it is a necessary component of economic designs of state policies. Understanding this dependence of the state on families to absorb the costs of care helps to contextualize how suffering in the present context of continued rapid social and political transformations will not ease. Further work on the anthropology of suffering will require renewed efforts to understand how social units such as the family instigate, experience, and manage disorder and disruption in their daily lives.

The different periods of training and philosophies of mental health have led to distinct generations of psychiatrists. The oldest group trained during the

1950s in the Soviet Union. The second group trained as general medical doctors first during the Cultural Revolution in the mid to late 1960s and only later specialized in psychiatry with exposure to Western theories at midcareer. The youngest group has been recently trained under the auspices of WHO financing or in the West at major research universities. Each of these generations has a different ethos regarding service and professionalism. All face lower status relative to other medical professions despite an initial boost in the 1950s, when there was a sense that Chinese mental health was very important. Presently, mental health care and promotion is secondary to psychiatric research, which focuses heavily on neuropsychology and pharmaceutical drugs. The hierarchy of power and funding has a direct impact on the ratio of patients to health workers at each institute and the amount of interaction with family members.

Psychiatric research in the People's Republic of China is of great interest to the WHO, primarily because it can provide such a large database of comparison. Chinese research focuses on four major areas: family and community studies, neurasthenia, psychopharmacology, and psychotherapy. Family research centers on the experiences of children and elderly patients, while community studies look at patterns of schizophrenia. Community studies are the specialty of Chinese mental health programs, as there is a heavy reliance on family care, especially for outpatient care. The Chinese interest in neurasthenia was sparked by Arthur Kleinman's (1986) work, which asserted that neurasthenia was a cultural category of depression. According to Sing Lee, neurasthenia is increasingly transformed into depression (1999). Psychopharmacological research has been conducted jointly with multinational pharmaceutical companies that either donate their products or produce drugs in China. An example is a project carried out in Xian and Shanghai by a Belgian multinational pharmaceutical company, that involved manufacturing drugs and carrying out controlled studies for dosage and effectiveness. Since the post-Mao reforms, a handful of psychiatrists have started to conduct psychotherapy in outpatient clinics for selected patients. Very few inpatients receive psychotherapy, however, as existing psychiatric services mainly attend to the severely mentally ill. In general, doctors deal less with common mental illnesses such as depression, anxiety, and psychosomatic disorders.

The physical setting of mental hospitals, especially the gates and walls of the institutes, is quite similar to other socialist entities, whether work units, factories, hospitals, or schools. Yet the stigma associated with the asylum makes the site particularly formidable to patients and family members. Like staff members, visitors become familiar with the grounds gradually. With normality as a goal of institutionalization, the subsequent process entails defining structure and transforming the daily life of patients. Socialist models of therapy in the post-Mao period still emphasize a liberation motif whereby individuals can be made into functioning citizens and workers again. And yet, within this process, personal meanings can be inserted into the spaces of the asylum. Even within the structure of daily life, there are multiple times and spaces within the clinics and wards that influence a person's experience of the asylum. The daily routines of inpatients are quite structured, while life in the clinical setting varies each day. Highly segmented spaces also define the subjectivity of the individual and the roles they have to assume in such spaces. Whether in the locked space of the inpatient ward, the nurse's station, the doctor's station, the fourth-floor administrator's office, or the activity room in the basement, all these rooms influence the experience of the individual.

During the 1990s rapid construction of new buildings, roads, and factories transformed the urban landscape into a modern socialist city worthy of the next Olympics. Hospitals were also part of the new construction. I returned to my institute in 1995 to find that the mental hospital had moved into a new seven-story building. The relocation to a new structure was symbolic of a renewed commitment to mental hygiene as a state enterprise. Whereas previously colleagues had all shared offices and patients shared large dormitory-style rooms, the floor plans now included private offices for physicians and researchers, while smaller groups of patients shared rooms. Nurses and other staff had a special observation room walled off by glass, similar to the panopticon psychiatric stations in contemporary U.S. hospitals. In response to my question of whether the remodeled mental hospital could be viewed as a new site of order and structured mentality, a psychiatrist remarked in confidence, "The building has changed, but the people have not." Administrators and health workers were excited about moving to new facilities, but in general the location made little difference to the subjects of the psychiatric state, the patients, and their family members. The same process of waiting for care and submitting to the order of the asylum is still the experience of those seeking psychiatric help. The engagement between social and political constructions of mental hygiene continues, and such notions are mapped onto the very structure of the hospital.

Recent intellectual and popular interest in psychology and psychoanalytic theory in post-Mao China has returned the focus to individual desire and ego. Previously banned, Freudian theories of sexuality became in vogue with the renewal of psychological theories. Street clinics specializing in psychotherapy opened for general practice on major thoroughfares in Beijing during the 1990s. NGO-sponsored mental health hot lines run in collaboration by medical professionals and trained volunteers have been operating in Beijing and Shanghai for several years. Several web sites devoted to popular psychology have also been started in recent years. Parallel to the public interest in psychology was the increasing use of psychiatry by the Chinese socialist state as means to achieve modernity. Lay public interests ironically intersected with official interests in the Deng reform era as both state and citizens began to explore the possibilities of private life and individual psychic interiors in the context of a radically transformed state government. While such a turn to private life could be interpreted as the return of the repressed, the drive to modernization has brought inevitable social changes for which many people are seeking panaceas. In the following chapter, I document the gradual involvement of bureaucrats and scientists as the number of qigong deviation cases in the psychiatric context grew and as the masters gained greater influence in the highest echelons of state bureaucracy.

CHAPTER SIX

MANDATE OF SCIENCE

THE MANDATE OF HEAVEN (*tianming*) is the Confucian notion that anyone who successfully seizes the reins of power has the rightful authority to rule over China. Over the centuries, many imperial rulers and their contestants have invoked *tianming* to declare each other as morally bankrupt while legitimizing their own form of hierarchy as better. In this chapter, I argue that the mandate of science operates as a particular formation in late socialism to anchor and legitimize state authority. Such a strategy offers state bureaucrats the opportunity to define themselves as modern protectors of ordinary people from the influences of evil (*xie*) cults and superstition. The alliance of officials with scientists also facilitates the embrace of expert knowledge as the basis of governmentality.

On December 9, 1999, television broadcasts on China Central Television (CCTV) showed President Jiang Zemin visiting the bedside of Qian Xuesen, renowned scientist and father of China's missile system, who was ailing and needed to be hospitalized. The following day, *Jiankang Ribao* (Health daily) and *China Daily* (*Zhongguo Ribao*) devoted their front pages to photos of this visit, much as they would have reported on the official reception of a visiting diplomat. The veneration given "Uncle" Qian reflected the status accorded Chinese scientists and how their projects are linked to the progress of the nation. How did scientists become such eminent state figures? Like medicine, science became integral to state formation and nation building especially during the socialist era. An engagement with scientific discourses is crucial to understanding the mobilization of allegiances among bureaucrats, scientists, physicians, and qigong masters in the formation of scientific qigong that would be politically correct and sanctioned. This chapter will examine the ways in which scientific discourses work in political contexts, especially as they relate to qigong. In the late twentieth century, the goals of Chinese socialist modernization relied heavily on discourses of scientific rationality and civilization that emphasized global economic dominance and docile, productive citizens. Science was embraced by both bureaucrats and qigong masters as a legitimating strategy for their own purposes.

Following Laura Nader's (1996) insight that an anthropology of science can reveal the boundary-making tendencies and ideological constraints of technoscience, my discussion will differentiate among the positions of several well-known masters, scientists, and officials. The roles of officials were ambiguous as they not only represented the state but also avidly participated in the practice of qigong for their own health-seeking purposes. Chinese scientists were far more outspoken about the need to define clear boundaries between authentic qigong versus the more contaminated category of pseudoscientific qigong promoted by masters. Policing the newly constructed categories would eventually coevolve with a state campaign for social order. Bureaucrats faced with forging socialist order in the post-Tiananmen period, framed by rapid transformations, were also aware that the fragmentation of social life and the appeal of multiple nonstate alternatives were spawned by economic reforms sponsored by the state. The emergence of unofficial players and cultural icons of power made the issue of defining political order, relying on scientific rationality rather than subjective knowledge, all the more important. Through science, bureaucrats reordered the classifications of qigong with scientists at the helm rather than qigong masters without scientific credentials. This chapter documents the renewal of scientism and the widespread application of scientific discourse in this process.

In the 1990s, a loosely organized web of government representatives became galvanized in a campaign for the regulation of qigong. Official state discourses about qigong began to be situated apart from popular qigong debates. While testimonial accounts of qigong healing continued to abound informally and in the popular press, state bureaucrats, through internal memos and state media, called for a differentiation between real (*zheng*) and false (*jia*) qigong. The goal was to separate out those individuals who claimed to be masters and healed for lucrative purposes from those with true abilities. The state-appointed bureau to regulate qigong invoked the new category of scientific qigong (*kexuede qigong*) as a means to cleanse and discipline the ranks of false masters. The category was quite porous and difficult to maintain as the criteria for true abilities differed greatly among laypeople and officials. For ordinary Chinese, the subjective experience of being healed was enough evidence of a master's abilities. For scientists and bureaucrats, however, double-blind tests, lab studies, and board examinations were deemed crucial to determining true abilities. The state and its representatives thus became crucial gatekeepers to control runaway popular perceptions of qigong masters. The oppositional boundaries created between true science and false practices or real qigong versus unscientific qigong were defined by bureaucrats rather than practitioners in order to regulate qigong as a state enterprise. Science and visions of what constitutes the modern life were an integral part of this construction. Even as charismatic masters and mystics were threatening to state order and not to be endured, qigong overall was nonetheless tolerated because the healing practice worked. Ordinary citizens and high-level cadres alike still sought masters for chronic ailments and still practiced themselves in spite of the new regulations.

Early anthropological analyses have viewed science and magic in several ways: as opposites, as a linear progression of social progress, or as complex categories of indigenous knowledge.[1] In spite of the state's attempts to separate the two, there was also an ironic intertwining of science and popular forms of healing. Qian Xuesen (a.k.a. Tsien Hsueh-sen), one of China's most prominent scientists, was frequently cited as one of the staunchest public supporters of qigong. Qian had studied physics in the United States and taught at M.I.T. and Cal Tech before he returned to China in 1955.[2] His knowledge of rocketry and aerospace science placed him in a leadership role, in touch with leaders such as Zhou Enlai and Mao Zedong. Over the past decades, he has received numerous accolades including State Scientist of Outstanding Contribution, the highest honor a scientist can receive in China. Many scientists and masters whom I interviewed mentioned in reverent tones how his support influenced the initial spread of qigong research. An article "Dr. Yan Xin on Scientific Qigong Research," prominently invokes Qian: "Professor Qian Xuesen has unequivocally advocated the creation of human body science. *At the same time, he predicted that the integration of Traditional Chinese Medicine, qigong, special human body functions, and a unified theoretical and scientific work will result in a great leap forward in medicine.* Furthermore he suggested that this event will revolutionize modern science as a whole, and that a second cultural renaissance will arise and come to fruition in China."[3] The patronage of China's premier scientist and the invocation of science by masters led to the privileging of science as a mean to measure the authenticity or power of qigong. In what follows I explore some of the concerns and debates that led to science serving as a form of "national consciousness" about modern life (Tang 1996, 23). Especially during the twentieth century, science represents a potent field of meanings in both the production of knowledge and subjects.

THE SCIENTIFIC SPIRIT IN
TWENTIETH-CENTURY CHINA

Notions about science and progress form a continuous strand linking imperial China and the contemporary socialist state. Joseph Needham's (1954–2000) multivolume history of Chinese science and civilization has established a tremendous legacy in the study of science. His evolutionary approach to science and technology proclaimed the importance to world history of ancient Chinese discoveries such as gunpowder, printing, and astronomy. Yet this master narrative also held that science and technology were static after the Sung dynasty and that any innovations emanated from the West as a result of industrial capitalism.[4] Debates about science and technology were central concerns in imperial China, particularly in the encounter with Western missionaries and diplomats. For instance, above the Jianguomenwai subway stop in Beijing lies the former observatory, complete with seventeenth-century astronomy instruments, of Father Matteo Ricci, the Jesuit priest who translated Western scientific texts into Chinese and became an imperial adviser to the emperor. Now a tourist attraction, the site is a silent reminder of how such instruments of scientific inquiry offered entry to imperial courts.[5] The binary opposition of the traditional sciences of China and the modern sciences of the West has been the subject of much consideration by scholars.

Instead of taking up Needham's question of why modern science did not emerge in China as it did in the West, my discussion examines how science became foundational in twentieth-century Chinese cultural politics. One reading suggested by Laura Nader is that "the politicization of science is unavoidable, not only because politicians, corporations, and governments try to use what scientists know, but because virtually all science has social and political implications" (1996, 9). How then can we begin to document the ways in which scientific inquiry becomes political? As Donna Haraway (1997) has shown, dual attention is necessary not only to understand the knowledge that is being produced but also to identify the invisible standards and categories that created such knowledge.

Lydia Liu's (1995) project of translingual practice, an "examination of language, discourse, and text" in the making of historical events, is particularly useful in understanding the formation of science in China. The term for science and its usage evolved in relation to debates about the philosophical aims of science. Before the contemporary usage of *kexue* as the nomenclature for science, *gezhi* and *gewu zhizhi* were more frequently used to connote scientific exploration. *Kexue* was a neologism from the Japanese term *gaku* and referred to the study of specialized subjects (Wang 1995). Wang Hui's study of early-twentieth-century scientists and scholars indicates that these terms reflected an underlying tension between the embrace or rejection of Western versus traditional Chinese science. Scientism and assumptions of social and national progress were promoted by intellectuals and new elites at the turn of the century. Contrary to C. P. Snow's assertion that science and the arts or humanities are two separate cultures, scientism and humanism been heavily intertwined in the formation of modern Chinese culture (Hua 1995). D. Y. Kwok offers a useful understanding of this framework: "Scientism, in general, assumes that all aspects of the universe are knowable through the methods of science. Scientism can thus be considered as the tendency to use the respectability of science in areas having little bearing on science itself" (1965, 3). Science has always been embraced by Chinese state leaders as a national platform essential for modernization. During the Republican era of the 1920s, attaining modern science, medicine, and technology was viewed to be crucial for the development of the modern state.[6] Usually the proponents of such notions of modernity were Chinese scholars who had been trained abroad, either in Japan or in Western countries, and foreign missionaries. In the first quarter of the twentieth century, May Fourth intellectuals interrogated the relevance of traditional values in light of China's place in the world. Chen Duxiu, a prominent intellectual, held that science could be a "replacement for Confucian values" (Wang 1995, 38). Even as the May Fourth movement could be characterized as "anti-Confucian" or "anti-tradition," according to Wang Hui, certain continuities such as the importance of science in the cultivation of the nation remained.

The construction of a modern nation occupied intellectuals well into midcentury. Under Mao, the problem of unifying the nation with scientific values rather than Confucian ethics continued. With the inception of the PRC, the socialist state continued to forge ahead with scientific progress as a national goal; however, the primary advisers were either Russian or Chinese scientists who had trained in the Soviet Union. Throughout the 1950s and 1960s, national progress was charted in terms of scientific progress guided by Marxist principles. Mao believed in the generative properties of science in building the socialist nation; scientists were regarded as an intellectual elite that needed guidance. Mao's vision of science, however, was far more "utilitarian" and localized than early modernizers' (Feurtado 1986, 4). The motto "Serve the People" quickly incorporated science to advocate the mass participation of nonexperts. Science for science's sake, with no immediate social function, was meaningless. Mao's policies also differed somewhat from earlier intellectuals' in the specific linkage of science with technology (*keji*) as a precondition to socialist modernization. During the early years of the PRC, many scientists were sent to the Soviet Union, while Russian experts were brought to China to promote scientific and technological innovations. Mao's science policy in the 1950s emphasized science as an "independent 'force of production' " that nonetheless required political consciousness and proper values by its practitioners 99). "Red and Expert" and "Walking on Two Legs" were common slogans during the Great Leap Forward. Such statements indicate the ideological role of science and technology as crucial to progress. The Maoist era solidified the relation between science and the development of the nation.

The post-Mao period opened with the National Science Conference, in which science and technology would become the cornerstones of modernization. Dengist reforms revised earlier interpretations of Marxist practice, such that scientific research could be disentangled from political debates to focus on applied industrial and agricultural development to "serve the economy and society" (Saich 1989, 17). During this redirection of science policy, concurrent debates about scientism and humanism were waged among intellectuals. According to Shiping Hua, three versions of scientism circulated during the post-Mao era: "The Marxist scientism of historical materialism, a Chinese style scientism of technological determinism, [and] the empirical scientism of systems theory" (1995, 6). Hua contends that three corresponding schools of humanism also emerged: Marxist, Confucian, and critical humanism. The schools differently engaged with questions of human nature and how Marxism could be used in policies of liberalism.

Scientists were among the first citizens to travel abroad in scholarly exchanges. They have continued to occupy prominent positions and are often viewed as spokespeople for the well-being of the nation. For instance, during the student demonstrations of the mid-1980s, a middle-aged physicist named Fang Lizhi became a visible figure who spoke out about concerns with corruption. While the international press focused on his alliance with student demonstrations and calls for democracy, Fang maintained a wide audience in China primarily because of his status as a scientist. After his departure to the United States, many other scientists within China continued to speak on national issues such as environmental concerns, population policy, and, more recently, market planning. During the 1990s, science and technology policy was readjusted from an emphasis on production to a focus on economic growth. This development required emphasizing basic research to enable new innovations (Yu 1999). Li Zhengdao, Nobel prize winner in physics, formulated the following metaphor to describe the importance of research and development in marketization: "Fish cannot survive without water and there won't be any fish market without fish. So when people try to develop a fish market they should, of course, prepare for more fish and, at the same time, a sufficient amount of water should never be neglected" (166). This metaphor sought to rationalize the limited goods that would result from shifting to market reforms.

The ethos of science as critical to nation building has pervaded most of twentieth-century China. Ann Anagnost (1997) notes that during the early twentieth century, intellectuals distinguished between material and spiritual development in the notion of Chinese civilization. Reformers in the 1980s maintained such a "split" but privileged material civilization over spiritual development (84). Science has been a critical part of this process. Scientific and medical qigong, for instance, emphasized the material elements of qi as a source of energy rather than the spiritual qualities of healing, which can be far too subjective. The use of scientific discourse to create new categories of real, scientific and false, unscientific qigong evolved after specific interest groups came together. Continued emphasis on scientism in the twenty-first century reveals how integral science and technology are to socialist modernization.

PSEUDOSCIENCE AND FALSE QIGONG

Qigong presented a critical tension concerning rightful authority between science and *mixin*. In order to combat superstition or pseudoscience, scientists vehemently opposed popular claims about the practice. If qigong was to promote a better life, then modern science was necessary to prove its reality and efficacy. Many masters, however, invoked science when claiming that their forms were sound. How would it be possible to combat pseudoscience when scientific discourse had already been appropriated in the popular context?

During the 1990s two movements were foundational to the state's containment policy toward false qigong: secularization and medicalization. Scientists took up the project of demystifying and secularizing qigong. Physicists were involved in empirical research to test the phenomena of qi. Publications in Chinese journals such as *Ziran* (Nature) tried to establish it as a physical element similar to wave particles. Another project, based at Qinghua University, involved experiments with masters such as Yan Xin. This process of secularization to take control of qigong discourse was closely related to the medicalization of qigong deviation discussed earlier in chapter 4.

The overlap between traditional Chinese medicine and qigong healing was further institutionalized. Several traditional Chinese medicine clinics offered qigong as a new addition to clinics. Yet the classification of qigong as a part of traditional Chinese medicine was not satisfactory to medical scientists, who were also bureaucrats of the post-Mao state. Masters with no formal training, who claimed to be able to cure anything, were still legion. Such healers were viewed as counter to the medical system, which was founded as a state institution on scientific principles. The medical bureaucrats wished to create order (*zhengli*) and distinguish between those healers who cured without formal training and those who were officially recognized by the state. Popular practices, such as mass healing lectures or practices in the park, began to be cast as *mixin* (superstition). Secular and medicalized versions of qigong, referred to as medical qigong, which reduced hallucinatory effects and removed the need for charismatic masters, were introduced. The move to medicalize qigong deviation and promote medical qigong was a key strategy to foster surveillance by doctors and licensed practitioners. Medicalization, according to Allan Young (1997), has always been about the assignment of symptoms and somatized disorders to routinized medical categories. Categorization has often been deeply politicized, as in the recently medicalized disorders of post-traumatic stress disorder (PTSD), chronic fatigue syndrome (CFS), and attention deficit disorder (ADD), among others.

Individual practices and magical claims about qigong in contemporary China existed within the same spaces that were created for post-Mao economic reforms and Chinese modernization. In the early 1990s, just when nostalgic Mao figures emerged as popular cultural icons and commodities, the term *mixin* also began to reappear. Mixin was a neologism borrowed from Meiji modernizers that referred to superstition or feudal thoughts during the early socialist era. The term was also used extensively during the Cultural Revolution (1966–1976) to purge heterodoxy. In the resurgence of state policy to contain qigong with superstitious overtones, there was an attempt to insert early Maoist socialist values to impose state order. In the ensuing battle to define clear lines between legal forms of qigong research and practice and more charismatic forms, mixin emerged as an effective rhetorical device with chilling resonances from the not-so-distant past.

In the second half of the 1990s a renewed form of scientism emerged. Discourses about pseudoscience would be used to distinguish practices that undermined the credibility of scientific knowledge and national progress from state-sanctioned forms of enterprises embracing the scientific spirit that cultivated the nation-state. The state sports federation figured prominently in the growing surveillance of healers. The charge of this agency was to prevent illegitimate healing practices by "corrupt" masters who only sought monetary gain. Internal articles documenting the fate of individuals who sought help with healing only to end bankrupt or with cases of qigong deviation were circulated among state agencies such as the Ministry of Health, the Public Security Bureau, and the State Medical Bureau. A formal public health campaign was initiated after more informal networking among these agencies.

The increased popularity of qigong and, by extension, masters of this art aroused several concerns in the state. First, the proliferation of informal social networks based on breathing exercises harked back to the days of the Boxers and other millenarian cults who in times of rebellion opposed the state. These groups often incorporated spiritualistic practices that involved immediate allegiance to a leader or master rather than any formal units of the party or state (P. Cohen 1997; Esherick 1987; Naquin 1976, 1981; Spence 1996). Examining the long history of rebellion and movements that challenged the mandate of heaven reveals that qigong shares powerful continuities with these early cults. Charismatic leaders, breathing exercises, and utopian views of a better future after the apocalyptic end of the regime were common to many such groups. But there were also some fundamental differences. Specific new technologies and changes in the transmission in the post-Mao era have meant that such practices tend to be urban based rather than originating among peasant groups in marginal regions. More women and literate individuals became practitioners, and, most significantly, the cosmopolitan travel of masters transformed such practices from village-based organizations to global empires.

Second, informal social networks helped to support the power of masters with little or no formal medical training to the extent that these individuals accumulated exalted wealth and prominence in the socialist market economy. Like rock stars in the West, these individuals had much charisma and garnered great attention and respect wherever they went. Rather than inspiring the polite clapping of official audiences, these individuals could move thousands to tears as they rocked to and fro in their chairs, convulsing with the power of qi. When Deng Xiaoping became party leader in the late 1970s, he sought to deemphasize the leader's role in hopes of avoiding problems with idolatry that had lingered after the chairman's death (and have resurged in recent years). The masters fed this desire for charismatic leadership after Deng's succession in the late 1980s. Their emergence depended on the renewal of the social sphere referred to as *minjian* (folk) that was nongovernmental and increasingly influential.

Third, a major consequence of these mass audiences was that people left the lectures feeling infused with the power of qi and ready to heal themselves or others. The sensations of *teyigongneng* (paranormal abilities) led many to perceive supernatural, even alien, entities impossible to control without extensive practice. When such individuals were brought into clinics of state medical institutions, the masters were accused of dabbling in superstition. From the perspective of the state bureau, it became necessary to call for regulation in a practice where *luan*

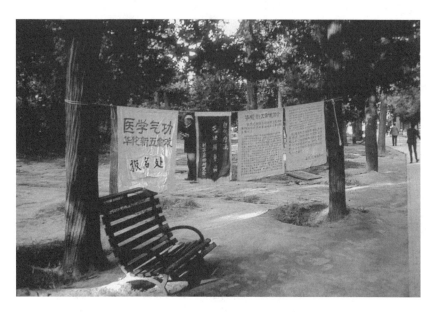

17. Banners proclaiming medical qigong in a Beijing park

(chaos) had taken over. Accusations of corruption and mixin were directed at specific masters who had amassed tremendous capital during mass healing sessions or in private.

The main concern of the state regulatory bureau was social order and morality. This required maintaining a fragile balance between modernization and meeting the material and social needs of the world's largest population. The unrest expressed in the Tiananmen demonstrations only furthered the resolve of the government to direct its attention to economic revitalization in an effort to quell popular protest over material disparity and corruption.

In 1989 a series of internal documents calling for the regulation of qigong began to be circulated among several state bureaus and ministries. Beginning in 1990, a few articles about deviation were published in major newspapers. It was not until the special summer conference at Beidaihe that a concerted public health effort began. The major newspaper that took part in this campaign against *qigong* was the *Jiankang Ribao* (Health daily). An overwhelming number of new cases showing up at Dr. Lin's clinic. Some patients and family members would travel several thousand kilometers from distant provinces in order to seek her medical advice after reading her articles.

The state regulation of qigong became even more aggressive in 1991. Private book stalls were raided by public security officers for any works that promot-

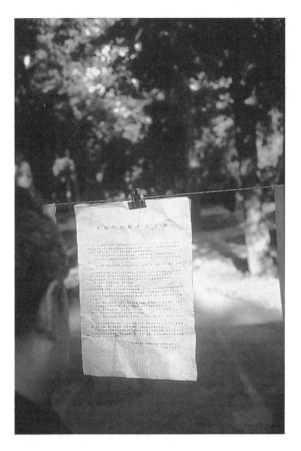

18. Announcement of medical qigong regulations

ed unscientific (*wu kexue*) or false (*jia*) qigong. As one state official told me, it was necessary to reduce the feverish interest in qigong (*jiangwen yidian*). Masters who wished to practice officially were required to register with the state qigong association. One could become licensed in several ways: by already having a medical degree and taking additional courses at a traditional medical school; by training with an officially recognized master; or by performing before a select board of officials and bringing in former patients to attest to one's healing powers. State authority was also inserted into the parks, in two ways: practitioners had to be formally registered members of an official school, and red and yellow banners appeared in parks stating what form was being practiced by a nearby group, along with the date of certification. Public security forces conducted regular raids on individuals who practiced without such banners. Practitioners of banned forms were taken in by local police to be questioned (see figs. 17 and 18).

The portrayal of masters or gurus as opportunistic or lacking in authentic powers can also be found outside of China. Han Ong's recent novel *Fixer Chao* (2001) has a central character who impersonates a *feng shui* (geomancy art of placement) master and gains access to well-off clients in the United States. Matt Groening, the creator of the cartoon *The Simpsons*, also produced a series featuring an entrepreneurial guru who dispenses advice with payment in advance.

CONTESTING RATIONALITY

The struggle for power and appropriate interpretations of qigong took place not just through scientific research but also in a more popular and accessible form of expression: the cartoon. In his analysis of the political life of cartoons and monuments in Indonesian politics, Benedict Anderson notes that "the cartoon appears to correspond history to the development of a certain type of consciousness—one that conceives of politics secularly as a separate, half autonomous realm of human interaction, and one in which mass publics share" (1990, 156). During decades of public art and politicized visual culture in socialist China, cartoons have been used to promote official messages of public health, moral campaigns, and daily life. Not surprisingly, just as scientific discourses were used to legitimate qigong, several cartoons appeared to question the legitimacy of such discourses.

In December 1990, an underground publication appeared in Sichuan Province featuring sardonic caricatures of bureaucrats who called for state control of masters and healers. The subversive publication was attributed to Mr. Yang, the young master in his early thirties discussed in chapter 3. The cartoons were taken very seriously by the Qigong Regulatory Council, which had by now coalesced into a vast system connecting the Ministry of Health, Ministry of Security, Public Security Bureau, military, and several research institutes.

The political cartoons intended to satirize how the state dealt with qigong healing. Many of the subjects that the cartoons ridicule—doctors, bureaucrats, and qigong masters—were sincere in their efforts to allay the suffering of patients and family members. The polemical nature of the cartoons stirred deep passions on both sides. Their content as well as the context of their reception ensured that a period of reckoning would follow.

In a rebuttal to news editorials that cast qigong as false practice, one cartoon illustrates how official newspapers were used to vocalize the views of the state.

Reminiscent of the slogans are pasted to walls during political campaigns, the word "*Gang zhong*" (Agitate) appears on a bucket of splashing ink. Nearby, one of the anthropomorphized newspapers, entitled *Kangfu Bao*, brandishes a megaphone apparently blaring "It is all false healing," a reference to frequent editorials with this message. The other figure, a paper entitled *Yongxi Bao*, carries in one hand a fan with the words, "Comrades, no need to look around," ironically indicating the lack of objectivity and willingness to see. This figure's other hand holds a menacing club emblazoned with the slogan, "Traditional Chinese and Western medicine criticize you," an acknowledgment that medical institutions were the force behind the snarling and unfriendly faces of the news editorials.

Scientists were lampooned for being impractical. Another cartoon is captioned, "Here is the real scientist." A person stands leaning forward, his neck stretched down and head buried in a sandpile, like an ostrich. His muffled voice states, "What is paranormal ability? It is all superstition." The sandpile is labeled "I am the only scientist," with a name at the bottom, spoofing the role of the leading scientist behind the secularization campaign. Rather than representing scientists as clear-headed visionaries, the cartoon points out the impracticality of their perspective on qigong and paranormal abilities.

Psychiatrists, too, were not immune from being satirized. In a third cartoon, a Daoist spiritual figure holds a spear over a woman standing on her hands. The caption reads, "The psychiatric specialist's abilities are now open. If I don't stop you now, no one will see the specialist." The skirt of the woman bears the label "Mental illness expert" while her shirt sports characters reading "Can see god," which happens to be a homonym for the name of the doctor who wrote the book on qigong deviation. In her upside-down state, the woman says, "What does opening the third eye mean? It's all qigong possession. Cure it quickly."

While physicians and scientists were spoofed as impractical, the bureaucrats who cracked down on private practices were portrayed as more threatening. In another cartoon, a medical official dressed like a martial artist is breaking signs while saying, "The more hospital signs, the happier I am. If I break these, the better I am." The sash around his chest reads "Medical official," and the sash hanging from his belt bears the name of an official. The various signs broken at his feet are for qigong classes, clinics, and research institutes. The cartoon referred to the closure of sites that did not become licensed and so were shut down by the state.

Officials are also spoofed in a fifth cartoon, which features an aging tiger dressed in cadre clothing and aiming an arrow. While "riding the tiger" refers to a popular folk image of power, here the tiger is portrayed as an overzealous but silly entity. The sign tied to the upturned tail states "Soldier of revealing qigong," followed by the name of the official responsible for targeting qigong groups. The caption reads "Turn against one group and speak against it so another may benefit," referring to the capricious nature of officials who indiscriminately created divisiveness among qigong associations.

Another cartoon shows a destitute figure representing a qigong practitioner holding a cracked bowl and pointing an accusatory finger at three newly established buildings that resonate with affluence and power. The caption reads, "All you newly rich from qigong are greedy. Life is hard, and I am jealous." The three new halls are named Sports Technical University, State Qigong Hall, and Scientific Sports Arena, referring to institutions that appropriated the practice of qigong as legitimate state enterprises. With official recognition, these newly minted institutions carry on lucrative business while the figure of the practitioner is forced to walk away, a beggar carrying an empty alms bowl. He stands on a wooden stick (an accessory of spiritual sojourners in the past), with the characters reading "True and Correct Qigong Method" at its upper left and the name of a master, Bai Shi, at the right. The cartoon is an indictment of institutions that profited from the regulation of qigong to the detriment of those who actually practiced authentic forms.

The underground criticism would not be complete without reference to the master who decided to go public with an exposé of power and corruption within qigong circles. In a final cartoon, a figure half in black and half in white performs as a magician. The caption reads, "It doesn't matter whether it is Eastern or Western, they will both help." On the table before him, the figure suspends a cloth over a bowl inscribed "False qigong." It is uncertain whether the bowl is about to be revealed or covered. The hat on the figure's head states "Magic tricks master," and his white mask bears Chinese characters that take on anthropomorphized features. It is clear that this figure is meant to evoke Mr. Ma, whom I discussed in chapter 3. The figure appears to be smiling, but the black half has a monstrous talon instead of a hand. The allusion is to the double meanings behind public statements, and the cartoon represents the master as a dangerous turncoat.

The cartoons reveal an alternate universe of interpretations and responses to the increasingly hostile environment for some qigong practitioners. But the unofficial publication and circulation of the images also signaled some bureaucrats to begin tightening the rein of control on qigong masters and the social disorder they engendered. Watchers outside China might ask, what could be the harm of a few cartoons? They were taken seriously for two reasons. First, they contested the value of state regulation. Secularization, via the licensing of masters and schools, incorporated qigong within the structure of formal authority. The medicalization of qigong and the pathologization of some forms as pseudoscientific contributed to the mandate of science as the rightful authority. Second, the presentation of such moves as self-serving and potentially ridiculous drew attention to the mobilized capital and networks of a master with a questionable reputation. Though it would appear that the state had initiated and implemented a damaging blow against pseudoscience and false qigong, the campaign would not have been possible without the involvement of masters. The move to regulate qigong mirrored the views of those masters who felt that the entrepreneurial promotion of miracles by some colleagues was going too far

Master Liu, the woman master in her midfifties, was outspoken about the need for scientific qigong, as I reported in chapter 4. Though she had been trained in the traditional way through the direct passage of knowledge from her father, who was a healer, she was concerned about contemporary forms of transmission. In her eyes, "Qigong needs to be controlled because it will go downhill from here. There are fewer and fewer people who understand it; we are all so busy. There are too many newcomers with very little *gong* [skill] who practice at a popular level and do a lot of damage. If patients try to give me money, I return it." Her views were amplified by Master Dong, who was slightly older, in his sixties, and had overcome cancerous tumors. He believed that qigong needed to be moral and develop a whole ethical system (*daode*) without money or hierarchy. Many other masters had differing views about the three *dashi* who became famous. Most of the masters I interviewed concurred that Master Zhen was indeed skillful and capable of healing. They were quite disparaging of Master Xu, however. With a disdainful sneer, Master Song tersely stated, "She deals with mixin, and *yuzhouyu* [universal language] is pure trickery."

The phrase "altered states" can refer to the different realms of consciousness that practitioners experienced. A second meaning plays on the image of a fragmented and dispossessed socialist bureaucracy that is also transformed by the social phenomenon. Innumerable high-level officials sought qigong healing as an alternative means to treat chronic disorders. Such engagement with alternative practices revealed the ambiguity between public roles and private lives in the post-Mao era. In the politicized Maoist era, private life and leisure time were required to mirror public identity. In the 1990s, even though cadres claimed to be private citizens seeking alternative health care, their association with prominent healers only confirmed the legitimacy of these masters. As in imperial times, the status of healers correlated with the status of their clientele. Usually, the acknowledgment of such relationships was by word of mouth.

CONFRONTATION BETWEEN THE
MASTER AND THE SCIENTIST

The debate as to whether qigong healing should have been regulated by traditional masters or by medical doctors became a much-contested issue. The battle for legitimacy between state-sanctioned scientific qigong promoting order and popular qigong healing crystallized in an unusual encounter between a master and a scientist bureaucrat. In the fall of 1990, Dr. Zhang, trained in TCM, published a series of articles denouncing the superstitious activities of masters who claimed they could heal any illness. His articles ended with an open challenge to any master who was willing to come forward and prove his or her healing abilities in an open confrontation (*dalei*). Weeks later, he was answered by Master Chen, a qigong healer in his midthirties, who wished to meet the challenge.

On a cold windy day in Beijing on November 30, 1990, the rational scientist met with the challenger. The bureaucrat had assembled a group of fellow doctors and scientists as well as leading journalists from various publications and media including Chinese Central Television (CCTV). All the figures ridiculed in the political cartoons were also participants. The master was accompanied by a handful of supporters, one man and two women. A total of seventy-five individuals, including myself, were gathered in a tiny room of the Academy of Traditional Chinese Medicine Research Institute. The room was arranged with tables assembled around the perimeter of the room in a large rectangle with a medical examination table in the center.

Dr. Zhang began by introducing himself and discussing the negotiations for the meeting. He held up a copy of the *Falu Yu Shenghuo* (Law and life) magazine containing an article of his asserting that merely the suggestion (*ansi*) of external (*wai*) qi could cure illnesses. He described how the response to this article had been quite angry: he started receiving threatening phone calls from masters who said they would confront him anytime. Master Chen sent a disciple to contact Dr. Zhang, leaving only an address in the old Western district of Beijing rather than revealing his work unit (*danwei*). Dr. Zhang then turned the table over to Master Chen. Wearing a black leather jacket and speaking in a thick Beijing accent, it was apparent that Master Chen was not part of the educated elite or bureaucratic power structure.

He began, "I cure many people, but they are only friends. I can cure one hundred illnesses but not one hundred people. I do not believe in ghosts."

Dr. Zhang interrupted and asked him, "When did you start healing?"

"About twelve or thirteen years ago," the master tersely replied.

"Do you incorporate medical theory in your healing?" asked Dr. Zhang.

"Yes, I begin with the meridians [*jin mai*], going from the twelve meridians to the twelve *gong guan*."

"What about your master? Did you have a traditional medical doctor or qi-gong master teach you?"

Master Chen smiled broadly and answered, "Both."

"What specific medicine did you learn from them?"

"Just the meridian theory." Master Chen continued to smile and wait.

"How old are you?" Dr. Zhang appeared uncomfortable.

"I am as old as I look," the master shot back.

"Can you cure someone and then let us ask you some questions?" Dr. Zhang continued.

"Only if you show me that you can cure someone, and then I will show you," Master Chen replied coolly.

The members of the audience started whispering loudly to each other.

A woman in her forties took the floor and spoke directly to Dr. Zhang. "You wrote that there is no such thing as external *qi*, but I have been cured by a master without being touched. What do you think about that? Explain your argument."

Dr. Zhang replied, "All those who study medicine know that to be cured partially involves ignorance and suggestion [*ansi*]. We need strict scientific research to understand what percentage of healing is due to these factors."

Another woman who identified herself as a physician responded, "We are all here to listen to both sides. We have to deal with patients in clinics. We do not want to disprove anything totally. We just want to see how you [Master Chen] cure and how we can do our job better. Can you please show us what we can do to understand qigong?"

Other members of the audience agreed, but before anyone could speak further, Master Chen stood up. "I am not here as a performing clown. If you want to cure someone, then do so. I know that I can cure for myself."

Three patients were brought into the room. An elderly woman in her sixties was helped by an attendant at each side. An older man was wheeled into the room by family members. A mother carried in an infant. The quiet of the morning meeting turned into a chaotic din as individuals all started conversations with their neighbors. Dr. Zhang stood up to readdress the audience, but few members were paying attention.

The elder male patient was diagnosed as having heart trouble and was laid down on the table. Dr. Zhang attended to the patient first, measuring his heart rate with a stethoscope. The patient quietly whispered details about his medical history. Master Chen then asked a few questions of the patient but suddenly slammed his fist into a table and shouted loudly, "How can I know if this patient is really ill!" By this time, most of the audience members had gathered into small huddles of conversation, paying little attention to the center of the room where the patient was lying. Much time was devoted to taking diagnostic tests using an electrocardiogram machine. The final announcement was shouted above the din, "There is no difference shown in the ECG."

The old male patient moaned and shouted, "I am here to be cured! I expected to be cured one way or another." His reedy voice was swallowed up in the general buzz surrounding him, an apt metaphor for all patients who sought qigong healing for relief of chronic pain only to be ignored in the social and political furor around them.

While the confrontation between master and scientist officially ended in a draw, a group of journalists continued to debate vehemently whether qigong healing was a matter of autosuggestion (*ziwo ansi*) or external (*wai*) qi. The audience by now had dispersed into small islands of debate, some people shouting at each other loudly to be heard; one heated debate in a corner nearly ended in a shoving match. People were quickly asked to disperse, and on leaving one journalist commented, "This was utterly meaningless. We came to attend a confrontation, but no progress was made in any direction."

A small-scale confrontation, parallel to the larger debate moments before, erupted between a woman journalist who practiced qigong and the male journalists, who were skeptical. As I watched the new altercation, I understood why press coverage on qigong varied across publications. Rather than being overwhelmingly dismissive or condoning of the practice as a profession, the personal stance of each journalist was reflected in his or her coverage of the topic. It was clear that the confrontation was directed to a broader audience beyond the meeting. If the media representatives could be convinced rather than officially commanded, as in an earlier ideological age, then the rational bureaucrat's task would be complete.

The containment of qigong by science revealed state projects of civilization such as the transformation of bodies into appropriate subjects. Steps to establish order (*zhengli*) in the social realm of qigong through science set the foundation for a renewed scientism that was much more public and widespread than earlier debates in the 1920s had been. New participants besides intellectual elites, such as qigong masters, ordinary practitioners, and their families, became involved. Mr. Ma, the former master turned investigative reporter and pseudoscience buster, devoted himself to public challenges of masters and healers who claimed to have extraordinary abilities. In addition to producing CCTV programs that debunked false qigong, he invited James Randi, an American magician and debunker of pseudoscience, to discuss tricks of the trade such as sleight of hand. Members of the Committee for the Scientific Investigation of Claims of the Paranormal (CSICOP), based in the United States, sent a delegation to China with the challenge that it would pay one million U.S. dollars to anyone who could prove his or her special abilities. The scientized version of medical qigong continued to be promoted, and in 1994 the State Council of China announced moves to strengthen science education.

Many practitioners and masters alluded to an apocalyptic ending of the present regime in the formation of a Great Universe. To understand this yearning for utopian nature and cosmos, it is important to remember the issues at stake. The orthodox socialist state's right to situate and confine the individual mentality is being contested by imagination that transcends official urban spaces. Qigong practice reveals how powerful and pervasive the Chinese tradition of healing and inner body cultivation can be. While remaining within the gates and walls of parks and city life, practitioners literally dissociated themselves from the state, acquiring power through breathing and visualization. Though the mind and body were intimately linked to the body politic, especially in politicized times such as the Cultural Revolution, in the post-Mao context qigong resituated agency within the social community and individual mind through altered states. The contemporary situation of qigong within the PRC remains distinct: defined by an ever-watchful yet ambivalent state eager to harness the popularity and power of qigong to the mandate of science and socialist modernization.

By the fall of 1995, it appeared that as popular interest in qigong subsided, new social practices of consumption such as buying videos, making calls on cellular phones, watching fashions shows, and redecorating the home became prominent. As Ms. Jiang, a former qigong practitioner and inpatient that I interviewed in 1991, showed me her remodeled living room and kitchen, where new linoleum covered formerly bare concrete floors, she talked about the transition to a life of material well-being. Between sips of carbonated soda, she reflected, "I don't practice qigong any more, not as often as I used to. I might [practice] once in a while, but there are so many things to do. Even though we have an extra day off on weekends now, my family and I are still much too busy. We are out working extra jobs or shopping all the time, making sure that we have bought items for the lowest prices because everything is so expensive now." Many qigong groups either disintegrated or practitioners adopted other forms of practice. According to Jiang as well as several scientists and doctors monitoring qigong, some groups merely shifted to more acceptable forms such as taiji or Buddhist qigong. Other individuals abandoned their practice altogether to pursue new pastimes such as *yangge*, a folk dance, or direct marketing.

While it appeared that the social world of qigong had receded, giving way to consumer life and the discipline of markets endorsed by the party, most charismatic leaders did not quietly retreat or become relics of the past. Though there was an immediate exodus from Beijing, the center of the secularization campaign, most masters were quite resourceful and relocated their quasi-empires to more favorable climes in the provinces and, more notably, abroad, where extensive networks of overseas Chinese and foreigners greeted them with enthusiasm. Such a move was predicted by all the masters I interviewed. Even with the regulation of qigong through science, most masters believed that the events in China were just the beginning and that "qigong will continue to grow." Tales of miraculous healing paved the way for several entrepreneurial masters to go transnational. Despite the reinforcements of scientization and medicalization to further the ideals of a socialist civilization, the flexibility and appeal of masters abroad led to the continued growth of qigong outside China.

CHAPTER
SEVEN

TRANSNATIONAL QIGONG

DURING THE 1990s qigong was a healing practice with few boundaries. It could be found in cities throughout Asia, the United States, Europe, and even Latin America. Rather than simply being a pan-Chinese phenomenon, with overseas Chinese as the sole practitioners, qigong became a transnational enterprise that was also taken up by non-Chinese of various backgrounds. Aihwa Ong's notion of the transnational as "situated cultural processes" rather than simply the movement of global capital helps to frame this discussion of the dynamic travel of qigong (1999, 17). In this final chapter I will examine the formations of social networks outside the PRC and the means by which masters attained tremendous followings both within and beyond China. I first describe the practice of qigong in Japan, Taiwan, and the United States, emphasizing how qigong masters were contemporary producers of Chinese spiritual healing. Turning to comparative fieldwork conducted in Taiwan over the summer of 1992, I discuss how individuals pursued their qigong healing and self-cultivation in different contexts. While in mainland China the practice of qigong became polarized into pseudoscience or politically correct forms, elsewhere it quickly became a global commodity with more spiritual overtones. In the latter half of the chapter, I will address the formation of *falungong* in relation to qigong. Examining the transnational characteristics of these two movements offers different ways to understand local meanings of practice. Moreover, such an analysis also challenges notions that transnational or global flows are solely about Westernization. Rather, the transnational flow of qigong also reflects the impact of regional influences and circulation.

Qigong masters were cultural agents active in marketing traditional or holistic medicine to middle-class consumers eager for alternative healing practices. Individual masters traversed the globe to hold mass healing sessions, teach foreign students, and create a wider base of capital and popularity. Such strategies followed capitalist contours of time and space, where market values and commodification shape local patterns of practice and association. Instead of informal groups gathering in a park to practice together, masters opened centers for instruction or healing and accepted payment for one-hour sessions, as do other branches of martial arts and traditional medical practices. Fee-for-service treatments were the norm. In tracing the fluid appeal of Chinese masters abroad, my central question is, how do these social formations of qigong differ from those in mainland China? I also examine why few cases of qigong deviation emerged in any of these transnational settings.

QIGONG FEVER IN JAPAN AND TAIWAN

I conducted comparative fieldwork in the cities of Tokyo, Taipei, and Kaohsiung (Gaoxiong) after completing fieldwork in Beijing. The availability of open space greatly influenced the configuration of practice. Even though Beijing had approximately eight million residents, with an additional million undocumented in the so-called floating population, the physical layout of the city includes former imperial sites as well as more socialist architecture.[1] The large number of urban parks and massive outdoor venues allowed most practitioners to practice outside, where the qi is reportedly better. In contrast, the sheer density of the population in the relatively smaller cities of Hong Kong, Taipei, and Tokyo meant that urban spaces available for recreational purposes were significantly fewer. Most individuals tended to practice inside their homes or at a qigong studio. Transmission of knowledge took place by instruction through masters and sometimes books. The commercialization of properties in these cities also made subtle differences in the perception of open space. In the PRC, because most property was state owned until the first half of the 1990s, residents practiced outside in every available area possible, referring to such space as state owned (*guojia de*) but publicly utilized (*gong yong*). In contrast, practitioners in other Asian cities tended to practice inside their homes or rented buildings to serve as private salons. Although it was quite simple for individuals in northern China to go to the parks for informal practice with others, practitioners outside the mainland had to go elsewhere. Rather than being readily accessible, practice tended to be elite and linked to the tradition (or lineage) of a certain master. One had to be accepted somehow, by induction and usually with payment, in order to continue practice.

My research in Japan was limited to one center during the winter of 1991. Though my visit to Tokyo was brief, the experience of finding qigong practice inside private studios was very informative. A Chinese bureaucrat insisted that I visit this qigong studio in north Tokyo. He had set up an exchange program after so many Japanese tourists had gone to China specifically to learn qigong. The center was in a semibusy commercial area on the third floor. I arrived in the early afternoon, slipped off my shoes, and awaited the center's representative, who was to meet with me. Over sips of green tea and with the aid of an interpreter, I was informed that Japanese interest in qigong corresponded to the number of Japanese tourists who had visited the parks in China. Many tourists videotaped practitioners in the parks and brought back books on the topic. Once back in Japan, they either found local Chinese residents who could instruct them or they made arrangements to return to China as students. In 1986 the Academy of Traditional Chinese Medicine made formal arrangements to have two masters sent to Japan as instructors and public lecturers on one-year contracts. All expenses were paid to the Bureau of Traditional Medicine in Beijing by the Japanese qigong associations. Practice emphasized gradual and regulated breathing exercises rather than the more charismatic forms. According to the manager of the north Tokyo qigong center, by 1991 there were over three hundred qigong associations with mostly Japanese students located in Tokyo, Osaka, and Kyoto. When I inquired as to whether there were any cases of deviation, the representative spoke without hesitation: in the five years he had been affiliated with the center, only one woman reported having hallucinations associated with qigong. She was a housewife in her midthirties who had taken up the practice for problems with neurasthenia. Regular treatment with the master resolved the problem, but shortly thereafter she stopped practicing altogether.

Our meeting ended with my receipt of a stack of printed information about the center, including prices for classes. After viewing the brochures, I understood that qigong practice in Japan required time and money, making it a more likely occupation for the wives of salaried men. The monthly charge for lessons was approximately $600 U.S. for two one-hour sessions each week. An overseas Chinese student later informed me that most Chinese living in Japan rarely went to such centers because they were so expensive. Occasionally a visiting master from China might offer a special lecture in Yokohama, where the majority of Chinese live. Their main focus, however, was on teaching Japanese clients in centers such as the one I visited.

I arrived in Taipei in the summer of 1992 curious to meet local practitioners and find out how common qigong deviation was. The summer air was hu-

mid and punctuated by the sound of urban traffic. I entered the gates of the
largest city park expecting to find dozens, even hundreds, of practitioners engaged in practice. Typical of most early mornings, there were martial arts
groups engaged in taiji or sword dancing. I wandered about the park expecting to stumble on qigong practitioners. Instead, I was dismayed to find neither
individuals nor groups practicing anything identifiable as qigong. This
prompted me to approach several people practicing taiji and ask whether there
were any qigong groups to be found in the parks. One middle-aged woman
shook her head while the other members looked puzzled. I rephrased my question, where can one learn qigong? The small group suddenly broke into animated discussion and suggestions. A man in his fifties said, "It's very simple:
just pick up any of the newspapers, and you'll find it all there." This was sec-
onded by another woman, who added, "It's all very fashionable [*liuxing*] right
now. There are lots of masters lecturing on qigong. You can find out about the
sessions in news ads. They're usually in large halls and gymnasiums at night.
Hundreds of people go and listen to a master while he or she gives off qi. It's
a very popular thing." In contrast to China, where newspapers were probably
the last places where masters would advertise their presence, in Taiwan qigong
practice was occurring in a context reminiscent of the mainland during the
1980s when it first became popular.

In his study on the formation of political communities, Benedict Anderson
(1983) describes how newspapers and other print media facilitate the flow of
ideas among communities. Print media, he argues, offer a forum that enables
political unity. Newspapers, magazines, and even cartoons offer a shared space
of imagined belonging and nation making. His analysis does not venture into
the privatized space of advertising, however. Ads can also be used to express the
sentiments of certain entities, including qigong masters.

In Taiwan, qigong masters occasionally ran ads for their services. In the early 1990s, this was the most common way to spread word about forthcoming
mass qigong sessions or the locations of regular classes. After reading several
advertisements in daily newspapers, I visited each site, hoping to find masters
and practitioners who could tell me more about local practices. The first school
I visited operated martial art studios where people could join as members and
train regularly. Photos of the master with various groups were plastered in the
hallway along with an honorary college certificate from an unknown American
college. (This was a common practice; photographs with famous people or cer-
tificates, especially from the United States, are a form of authentication for
masters.) When I observed the classes, over 90 percent of the students were
male, and the emphasis of the practice was on external (*wai*) gong and enhancing male vitality. As a woman, I found it difficult to gain access to the

master. I was told that only those of his disciples (*tudi*) who had studied with him a long time could ever see him. Several weeks later, however, a male European American student who wished to find out more about the practice was able to gain an immediate audience.

I left the studio in search of other masters. As I visited one qigong school after another, I soon realized that the practice did not take place outside in the parks because most masters wished to maintain their art as a private pursuit and source of income. Many studios took on the aesthetics of the specific form that the master espoused. Some studios were like large martial art arenas, where students were expected to join a class. Other sites were primarily clinics, where individuals with chronic illnesses or other ailments could seek treatment.

At the Academia Sinica, a qigong instructor held special lessons for scholars during the lunch period. Normally, Mr. Tseng was the grounds and maintenance person for the academy, but during lunch hour the roles reversed, and the scholars addressed him as *sifu* (the local pronunciation of *shifu*, master). When I interviewed him about his practice, he told me he had been practicing an indigenous Taiwanese form of cultivation through breathing for over twelve years. I asked whether qigong fever in mainland China had any influence on practice in Taiwan. His reply was startling and yet made much sense. "Qigong is hot [*re*] everywhere, but the books and information that we get about it don't come directly from the mainland but from Japan. It's even bigger in Japan than it is in Taiwan, although qigong is quickly becoming popular here, too. People here don't look to the mainland as a model; they look to Japan." I returned home, passing official buildings and small streets reminiscent of Japanese suburbs, with a renewed realization of how much Japanese influence still lingered in urban Taipei.

The local English newspaper had an ad for qigong lessons that indicated the master was seeking foreign students. I visited the studio, located on the twelfth floor of a large office building. In contrast to the gray, official exterior of the building, the studio inside resembled a Buddhist temple, complete with incense and sounds of chanting. (Later, I found the chants were played from an audiotape that was available for purchase.) The master sat at a table and greeted me calmly. He agreed to let me use his studio as an ethnographic site, especially as he was familiar with the social issues related to qigong in urban Taiwan. His shelves were lined with clippings and books on the topic as well as Bataille's *Inner Experience*, which documents the author's mystical experience. It was clear that this master was quite cosmopolitan, blending old with new. He called himself Michael and incorporated the latest medical technology in his practice. When clients came in for an initial diagnosis, he would use an electronic pulse-reading device linked to a computer, which would produce a printout to interpret. His regular students included Taiwanese and overseas Chinese as well as Americans and Europeans. Yet there was an element of traditional Daoist practices in his work, which emphasized deep breathing techniques and internal alchemy. I accompanied the master on several excursions. Once, he was asked to purify a home using geomancy, or fengshui, to exorcise a young child who could no longer sleep. In another "new age" experience, I accompanied Michael and his assistants to the Taiwan Cement Corporation, one of the most wealthy and powerful companies in Taipei. In the main conference room, a large round table in the center, the senior executives gathered twice a week to practice qigong with the master. As loud burps and other bodily sounds punctuated the air, together with deep breaths, the structure of the master-client relationship seemed to be overwhelmingly similar to the mainland, where qigong masters also fostered intimate relations with powerful clients. In Taiwan, however, qigong was a commodity only available to those who had the time and money to learn it in a private setting.

There was little use of qigong deviation as a psychiatric category outside the PRC. This was due not only to the smaller number of practitioners but also to the fact that the phenomenon is limited to those who practice under the supervision of a master. I inquired at the state psychiatric institutions and interviewed psychiatrists in Taiwan as to whether there were any incidents involving qigong deviation or possession. A few psychiatrists had heard of the disorder, but all the cases of mental illness in their institutions corresponded with the DSM-IIIR. Most psychiatrists noted that the presence of active temples in the urban setting meant that a number of psychosomatic cases or culture-bound syndromes were dealt with in the community rather than reaching the psychiatric clinics. Jung-Kwang Wen (1990), a psychiatrist and ethnographer, has written an account of one such temple in southern Taiwan. Members of the Dragon Metamorphoses Hall regularly experienced trance and possession as part of spiritual practice. Rather than being viewed as deviant behavior, the experiences of followers were deemed normal as long as they stayed in the temple and did not transgress into ordinary life. Dr. Wen believed that such places provided important spaces for spiritual healing, such that mass qigong sessions were not as unique in Taiwan.

QIGONG NETWORKS IN CALIFORNIA

I documented the social development of qigong practice in North America, primarily California, from 1994 to 1999. Qigong appealed to two specific audiences: local Chinese communities and followers of alternative healing. As in the PRC, qigong in the United States initially was part of the spectrum of martial arts such as taiji and wushu. Most major cities with these communities also had qigong masters who had established themselves as teachers and healers. As in Japan, popular knowledge in the United States stemmed from various sources but primarily from tourists who had been to China or those who had sought qigong healing for chronic ailments. Chinese-language newspapers and new age publications frequently included articles on the topic, relating the practice to cures for chronic back pain, stress, and even AIDS. The active exploration of qigong in the United States can be as belonging to a larger social and political context where alternatives to biomedicine are sought.

The growing networks of masters abroad correlated with the growth of healing communities in the United States. When I returned to Berkeley, California, in 1991, Dr. Zheng, one of the three famous masters in China mentioned in chapter 3, was concluding a coast-to-coast tour in the United States. While in China, Zheng traveled to various work units that sponsored his marathon lectures, some lasting five to six hours. In the United States, he drew on local communities of Chinese intellectuals and businesses. Interviews with his sponsors indicated that he had a vast network in the United States, an association that included major Chinese community leaders as well as individuals whom he had healed and who thus became willing patrons. Advertisements in Chinese newspapers and at local acupuncture centers announced his arrival in the Northern California Bay Area. In May 1991 he held a large session in the Masonic Temple of San Francisco. Posted at the entrance was a warning that participants would be held responsible for their own actions, alluding to possible physical reactions and trance states that could occur later. The handwritten sign stated the following:

Important announcement

1. We do not accept persons who are actually ill but they could ask their relatives to listen for them to have a transferable effect.

2. During Dr. Zheng's emission of qi the sensibility of each person's reaction is quite different. In case of any eventuality, each person must take the responsibility for oneself.

3. Please be seated on time and don't leave your seat at will.

The audience was largely composed of members of the local Chinese American community, immigrants as well as second- and third-generation Chinese. Students, clerical workers, small business entrepreneurs, and professionals were part of the mixed constituency of Chinese and Americans in the audience. Similar to such gatherings in China, several individuals who were incapacitated were pushed in on stretchers or wheelchairs. A handful of European Americans was present, and a translator was on hand. Dr. Zheng began his lecture by describing qi and the power of qigong. Various individuals with backgrounds in physics or medicine were called on to give oral testimony to his abilities. Members of the audience gradually began to sway and moan during Master Zheng's hypnotic lecture. The collective mood was electric, with members erupting with sudden cries and swaying back and forth in their seats. Some shone with ecstatic smiles of delight; others shook with deep, heavy sobs. The lecture brought together people of various backgrounds and ethnicities in search of a common goal: self-healing. As in China, the master's discussion lasted over five hours, during which he discussed the difference between internal and external qi. As some individuals ran up and down the aisles, moved by the power of qi in their bodies, Zheng calmly pointed out that these people were more sensitive to the powers of his qi and that this was a natural response. The finale came with a demonstration of his practice where he externalized his qi. Suddenly, the audience erupted into mass emotional frenzy. Various audience members started to moan softly or uttered loud primordial sounds. But, a consummate master, Zheng knew how to bring the participants back to calm. The response of the audience indicated that cultural practices traveled and gained value as masters themselves became the currency for alternative healing communities.

Special lecture tours were not the only way masters gained legitimacy or built their followings. Such events were coordinated by volunteer networks of students or patients. On an institutional level, however, growing numbers of masters opened private clinics, while schools of traditional Chinese medicine and holistic institutes sponsored masters to give lessons. In the fall of 1997, the Second World Congress on Qigong, entitled "Qigong: Inner Power, Vitality, Longevity for Self, Family, Organization, Community, and the World," was held in San Francisco, the first meeting in the United States. The program brochure opened with proclamations for Qigong Week in San Francisco by the city mayor and even greetings, accompanied by a glossy photograph, from the president of the United States. Sponsored by the East West Academy of Healing Arts and several dozen other institutions, the three days of plenary sessions, master workshops, performances, and exercise sessions offered a wide range of topics specific to qigong. Sample papers, among the forty-six presented, included "Peak Performance in Corporate Health," "Qigong and the Immune System," and numerous clinical reports on the rehabilitative effectiveness of various forms. Attendance fees ranged from $315 to $495 on a sliding scale. The presence of several hundred participants signaled a coming of age for qigong in the United States.[2]

MY DISCUSSION THUS FAR has primarily described the different contexts in which qigong thrives as a popular alternative to biomedicine and even traditional Chinese medicine. The experience of charismatic healing was similar in all contexts, but the location and configuration of power was different each time. In the PRC, parks and other public venues figured prominently. With the growing insertion of state regulation, certain forms of group practice went underground. In Taiwan and Japan, qigong was more of a private enterprise, a means of spiritual practice and healing with a price tag. In the United States, too, qigong was initially a private enterprise dependent on social networks that operated coast to coast. To practitioners of Chinese descent and other ethnic backgrounds, the practice provided traditional healing that relied on the internal power of the master. Most masters marketed and emphasized the mystical and holistic aspects of the practice to fit it within the American paradigm of Asian medicine. The travel of masters was crucial to the expansion of their schools and reputations. In a cultural feedback loop similar to that experienced by Chinese artists, attracting clients and patrons overseas could lead to ultimate legitimacy and social capital at home in China.

MASTERING NETWORKS

The notion of networks, which facilitate the flow of information, is particularly useful in understanding how masters managed their transnational followings.[3] In China, most masters and healers tended to have networks within the social structure of a knowledge base limited to their students or patients. Only a handful of masters were able to amass wider patronage networks across the country. Still fewer were able to parlay their networks into major enterprises. How do qigong networks in a transnational context differ from those within China? At first glance, it would seem there would be a world of difference. Qigong masters abroad and in China, however, relied on very similar strategies of propagation. The primary basis of developing a following was not monetary capital but social capital. Qigong masters visited former patients or followers abroad and could be busy healing supplicants just from this first ring of relations in immigrant and transnational Chinese communities. The second circle came after opening a school, association, or clinic in a different part of the country. Here, friends, relatives, neighbors, and coworkers of the inner circle could receive instruction together on a regular basis. The third circle came after a lecture circuit was established. Touring regions or countries with open events was the ultimate public relations promotion. Books, tapes, and videos of a master could generate income in addition to attracting larger audiences.

Commodification of qigong practice within China took place to varying degrees. Initially, one might be able to purchase, for a small fee, books and tapes about a particular form of qigong. Depending on the master and school, tickets could be purchased to attend a special public session or perhaps arrangements could be made for a private healing session. Most practitioners and masters alike stated a sincere wish to create a better world rather than to accumulate capital. Even so, many followers attracted to a particular master still brought with them the flow of funds in exchange for healing. One well-known master opened a qigong center in Shandong Province atop a hill that followers referred to as Mount Lotus. Originally an undeveloped site, within a decade the location was transformed into a miniature city and tourist attraction with hotels, restaurants, shops, supermarkets, and a qigong clinic that local and national dignitaries as well as believers could visit. In addition to a glossy book published to celebrate the first decade, videotapes and web sites were available for practitioners to view. The success of such places depends on the style of the master. In order not to appear like a shyster, cult leader, or promoter of false qigong, such masters adopted official chic by wearing the clothing of cadres, downplaying consumerism, and emphasizing officialness with red seals. Prominently displayed photographs of state officials or scientists visiting the center also lent a sense of approval.

Patronage of masters abroad was crucial for operation either as a lecturer or healer. A master, however, also needed to overcome difficulties with language and networking in the American setting. In the fall of 1993, I was invited to a special qigong conference at a Los Angeles suburban college. I presented a scholarly paper on qigong deviation, expecting the audience to consist primarily of academics and China specialists. To my surprise, there were many more individuals in the audience of over two hundred who were suburban upper-middle-class anglos drawn to attend because of their practice. Master Tu from Henan Province had left China in 1990 and quickly established himself within the academic community. When he lectured about the powers of qi, the audience swayed back and forth, recalling Zheng's performance in San Francisco. It was overwhelming to witness how a cultural practice such as qigong could translate and cross social and political boundaries. When I interviewed one Caucasian participant in his fifties about his physical responses, he said, "Master Tu's qi is very powerful. I could sense every ounce of qi that was emanating from him to me. It's helped my asthma and back problems tremendously. Even some of my hair is turning dark again." To him, it was clear that the practice of breath work and meditation was effective. Ultimately, a master's reputation relied not so much on wide networks but on whether his skills were convincing enough to his patients and clients.

While so far I have focused on the entrepreneurial activities of male masters, women masters have also created prominent qigong networks in the United States. Master Sima, who was Vietnamese but resided in Taiwan, promoted a meditative, trancelike form that swept Vietnamese and Asian American communities throughout the United States. More locally, Dr. Zheng, a Chinese American biologist who specialized in cancer research for twenty years, opened a special retreat center in Santa Cruz called the Land of Healing Buddha. The retreat emphasizes self-healing through training in qigong practice; its clients are primarily middle- and upper-middle-class Americans who are willing to try alternatives, particularly new age forms, to biomedicine. Master Chow, another local qigong healer in the Northern California Bay Area, opened a healing center in 1977 and has been teaching specific forms of qigong exercises. Master Qin, a master in her forties, learned meditation and healing first from her grandmother and then from a Buddhist nun at a well-known temple. Initially an academic in China, she came to the United States to attend the Second International Congress on Qigong in 1999. Since then, she has opened her own qigong school and operated special workshops. Along with maintaining a web site, she offers special fasting seminars, which involve a variation of *bigu* (deep meditation and fasting), to mostly non-Chinese students in the Bay Area.

VIRTUAL QIGONG

The phenomenal development of the Internet as a conduit of information for vast numbers of interest groups and as a lucrative means to reach new markets created unique spaces for qigong practitioners and masters to connect. In 1994 I conducted a Web search on qigong to see whether there were any sites devoted to this topic. To my surprise, there were several hundred. Over the years, the number of sites has increased geometrically from several thousand to over tens of thousands depending on the search engine. Practitioners could engage in dialogue on special list servers and chat rooms. Participants on one list from which I received emails for nine months daily raised questions similar to those in China. Members often addressed the history or moral philosophy of the practice. Even more frequent were questions about the experience of qi and subsequent relations of one's qi to the environment. In 1999 it was not unusual to find personal narratives similar to spiritual conversion stories available on the Web. "Before" and "after" photos of individuals diagnosed with terminal cancer, victims of near-fatal accidents, or people battling with weight problems accompanied the compelling narratives of healing. These narratives were close replicas of the miraculous qigong healing stories that I encountered firsthand in parks and hospitals in China. For individuals with online access, the Internet facilitated unprecedented access to new realms of communication and the production of knowledge.

The travel of masters and more recently the circulation of their teachings beyond China have meant that old rules of licensing and containment are no longer effective means to control the spread of charismatic forms of qigong. Masters who were wired to flexible formations of capital and technology could gain access to new spaces and audiences. Such extensions of their organizations required timely and devoted maintenance by staff or volunteers to create and update web sites. The development of qigong groups without boundaries or regulated social spaces thus went beyond the reach of the nation-state. The virtual locations of some groups were represented by Web addresses, which replaced the signs posted on street posts or corners of busy intersections.

CULTIVATING BODY POLITICS

In this final section, I trace the development of one cultivation group, *falungong*, which the Chinese government declared an evil cult in 1999. The word *falun* refers to the wheel of Dharma, while *gong* is the same as in qigong. Many practitioners also call it *falundafa*, in which *dafa* translates as "great method." I use "falungong" (FLG) to refer to the organization as this was the term most frequently used in China and by its membership. During the 1990s its founder, Kung, began to lecture and set up teaching stations in northeast China.[4] Like other qigong practitioners, most falun enthusiasts said that an interest in healing was their main reason for starting practice. Followers also found the emphasis on self-cultivation and spiritual well-being appealing. The amalgam of qigonglike exercises with Daoist notions of cultivation and Buddhist symbols seemed familiar and provided quick relief as well as an instant community.

Kung and his organizers utilized certain strategies to achieve rapid growth. First, in contrast to most qigong classes in China, which charged fees, all classes were free to interested parties, though lay practitioners still purchased books or tapes. Once practitioners became regulars, they were encouraged to spread the news about self-cultivation and to bring in new members. This emphasis on expansion was perhaps the main reason for rapid dissemination. Eventually, an elaborate web of practice sites, instruction centers, teaching centers, branches, and city or provincial headquarters was established (Wong and Liu 1999, 25). The group was possibly one of the largest organizations to have emerged in the 1990s, though estimates by the government (2 million members) and by the group (100 million) widely differed. When I returned to China in 1996, many of my colleagues mentioned this new form of qigong to me. Established bookstores and small book carts throughout Beijing sold Kung's text, *Zhuan Falun*. It seemed that he had followed the path of other masters who became entrepreneurial.

Falungong became rapidly established outside China as well. In 1996 Kung moved to Flushing, New York, where he continued to promote his form of self-cultivation and healing, initially to the Chinese immigrant community.[5] Lessons were promoted not only by word of mouth but also via the Internet. Rather than maintaining its presence as an internally closed unit, the group spread information about representatives and practice sites to any interested parties. Despite the claims by followers that falungong was not an organized group, the numerous web sites with names and telephone numbers of local practitioners in cities across the United States, Canada, Australia, and Europe indicated impressive networks and organizational form.

Falungong initially competed for membership with other qigong groups when it first emerged both in China and the United States.[6] The practice spurred debate among qigong practitioners. When I was a member of one qigong list server during 1996–97, an email debate offered some revealing distinctions about the new form. On January 26, 1997, a qi list serve member sent out the following query, "Has someone answered the question about why falungong practitioners are excluded from qigong practice? A couple of people here on campus asked, and I don't know the answer." A handful of fellow practitioners quickly replied and mentioned how their master believed the forms were not mutually exclusive but that it would be better to practice different forms at separate times of the day. Two members gave more extensive commentary on the differences between their school of qigong and falungong. I have included the texts with original syntax and spelling without grammatical corrections to retain the voices of the writers. My interpolations appear in brackets.

The first response frequently invoked the adherence to science as crucial for the development of qigong.

Hello Everyone,

I believe lots of local chapters have got some loses [losses] affected by FA LUN GONG. It is not BAD at all] Zheng's can only attract some people who believe QiGong should go the Science & Research way, not the religion way.

From what I have experienced, FA LUN GONG is a religion instead of QiGong. In fact the founder emphasize that FA LUN is not QiGong at all, it is FA(LAW). FA LUN can not combined with QiGong easily. FA LUN GONG claims all other QiGong are at least low level, most of them are evil. The founder, Mr. Kung is the highest level master(Higher than Jesus, Budda . . . It is OK for FALUN followers to believe what they believe . . .

One extreme example of FALUN GONG is that people should not take medicine after they practice FALUN. Lots of naive people in China practiced this OUTRAGES rule and paid their life price. (My friend told me that they are lots of BAD examples happened in China by FALUN, two of people he knew, one was dead and another become a plant people [vegetable].

My point is that Qigong characterized itself as Science oriented, we want to explain everything through science, at least science attitude.

Everything in science are measurable. Measurement is the KEY for QiGong to become science.

Science currently cannot measure Qi, (de)virtue, relaxation, quietness, love . . . But we can measure some of the QiGong by-product: How long a people(with certain position) can practice QiGong; How heavy, far away a person could use his/her Qi power to push a foreign object; How long a person can endure a BiGo [Bigu] state; How deep a person can see through a covered object. . . . .

If we can set up a qualify testing committee to verify people's Qi power by his/her by-product capability, that will be an important step for QiGong to go to science. So at least we will know some people are level 1, 2, 3 . . . Right now all the high level QiGong friend I know are too humble to be scientific.

I wish I had the money to sponsor this committee.

Long before the Chinese government's opposition to falungong, this commentator asserted his belief that FLG wasn't qigong but a religion. Moreover, concerns about the effectiveness and negative outcomes of this form were raised. Science was invoked as a crucial measure for authenticity and to verify whether new forms could really heal.

The second respondent also emphasized how falungong was more of a spiritual group than one focused on promoting the practice of qigong. Unlike the first commentator, the second writer was in a more compromising situation because his parents were deeply involved in falungong.

My parants practice FaLun and are indeed coodinates for one group, they sent me books and are trying to make me practice Falun, too. But from the book and what they told me, Falun is indeed too extreme for my taste. One example is that their master Mr. Kung said that most qigong masters are just evil spirits of foxes attached to human body. Educated in modern science and believing in that people should respect any belief, I can not accept this at all. I would agree that Falun is indeed a religion.

However, one can always learn from anything, hence Falun should have something worth learning in it. The problem is that Falun is very exclusive, if one really want to practice it, one must give up all other methods including Tai Chi. One story told in the book is that: a student of him once saw the Fa3shen1 (law-body, a special term, I don't know exactly what it means) of Mr. Kung coming, he was very glad and ask Mr. Kung to come in, Mr. Kung's Fashen said that his room was too messy and left. The student realiezed later that his room was full of all kinds of qigong bookks, he burned and sold all of these, then Mr. Kung's Fashen returned again. (*Zhuan FaLun* P215).

I read these books ocassionally, but I make up my mind that I only learn from it, and I won't become a real Falun practitioner.

On the one hand, falungong emphasized breathing exercises, meditation, and movements similar to standard qigong forms. Some qigong practitioners even managed to practice several forms including falungong at different times of the day. But focusing primarily on spiritual cultivation through the turning of the wheel of Dharma, the icon that looks like a backward swastika, was quite different from concentrating on qi energy. Followers were told that the wheel spun in the air or within one's belly to promote healing.

On an organizational level, the group was very media oriented and savvy about its public presentation. Each cell or practice site had a volunteer spokesperson and organizer. Such individuals were ordinary practitioners who had been recruited to gain more members. Regular "experience-sharing" conferences, in which new and experienced followers described how they were healed and how their lives were saved, took place across the United States. Rather than emphasizing the power of the master through qigong performances and then public healing with supplicants, the power of healing narratives took center stage. A whole day would be based on testimonials of followers who claimed to be healed by their master and the wheel of law. Member after member would get up to share his or her healing story, read aloud from scripted pages. Organizers also devoted much effort to petitioning municipal offices across the United States to recognize Kung officially as a special guest. Proclamations of Mr. Kung Day were declared in cities such as Chicago, Houston, San Francisco, among others.

Beyond these activities, falungong stood out for one primary reason. In China, whenever any negative criticism was publicly raised about the sect in the form of news editorials, published articles, or televised programs, protests by followers often followed. Though hundreds of qigong masters and forms circulated in post-Mao China, only one other qigong master had overtly criticized the state through lampooning bureaucrats (discussed in chapter 4). The falungong organization was the only group that resorted to surrounding media offices with dozens sometimes hundreds of protesters. A foreign correspondent for the *Washington Post* noted in July 1998 that several dozen falun followers had protested in front of the Beijing Television Station building after the broadcast of a show warning of the dangers of qigong (Laris 1998). The continued mobilization of followers to contest institutions and bureaucrats offering negative views about falungong began to resemble eerily what Susan Naquin has noted about millenarian rebels in China's past: "It was in this way that the eight trigrams were created. Vigorous leaders had used ordinary sect ties to build a sect organization of extraordinary size and scope, and they emphasized one dimension of the religion—its vision of apocalypse and millennium—to mobilize believers into rebellion" (1976, 117). In a different context, David Ownby noted a "language of mobilization" that was utilized by followers of the Way of the Temple of Heavenly Immortals in Henan province during the early Communist era (1940s–1950s) (2001, 87). Such actions would transform falungong followers, who initially sought healing and self-cultivation, into a political organization seeking legitimacy that has come to plague the Chinese leadership.

On April 26, 1999, falungong became front-page news in the international press when an estimated ten thousand members staged a silent protest outside Zhongnanhai, the official state compound where leaders reside. The timing of the event, on a Sunday in the spring when several key historic moments of the twentieth century are remembered such as the May Fourth movement, the tenth anniversary of the Tiananmen protests, and especially the fiftieth anniversary of the People's Republic of China, meant that the demonstration drew the attention of an already primed foreign press waiting to hear of any demonstrations or acts of protest. The location of the gathering also made clear the intentions of the group and the significance of this public act. Had the followers assembled in a park where qigong practice is regularly practiced and accepted as a daily event, few people outside the city would have ever heard about it. Instead, holding the protest in front of the official compound where state leaders reside took many, including the military guards, by surprise. "How could so many people gather without notice?" "Do they really have that many followers?" were questions asked by many journalists. Eyewitnesses from the scene indicated that the thousands of protesters, mostly in their forties through sixties, lined up silently in orderly rows while designated appointees spoke with onlookers or reporters. Without the usual signs, banners, and slogans expressing demands, even public security officers were hesitant to start moving the crowd, which easily outnumbered them. Residing in the United States, Kung claimed to have nothing to do with the protest in Beijing. His organization and the protesters that day, however, demanded a meeting with Premier Zhu Rongji and a retraction of an article published in the *Tianjin Qingnian Kexue Bao* (Tianjin youth science and technology journal) that warned about the dangers of cults. The protest directly confronted socialist leaders, which granted far more visibility and infamy than even perhaps what its organizers had hoped to achieve.

THE STATE STRIKES BACK

The organized rows of middle-aged and elderly dissenters outside the state compound gates of Zhongnanhai presented a disturbing sight not merely for their large numbers. These were not impulsive youths in their twenties, as had been the case a decade earlier. Instead, the protesters came from the backbone of Chinese society. Many of the older participants were contemporaries of the leadership who had undergone the same formative experiences of nation building and sacrifice. Their presence before the state compound indicated rifts beyond claims of misrepresentation in the media. The protest on April 22 was declared illegal. When more FLG practitioners showed up to protest, there were swift actions taken to round up any demonstrators immediately. International media portrayed the tearful removal of mostly middle-aged women and elderly. Despite rough handling by police and soldiers, the demonstrators performed acts such as cleaning up or offering water to their captors. These images resonated with coverage of student demonstrators a decade before. It appeared that foreign press and falun protesters were equally eager to demonstrate similarities between the protests of 1989 and 1999.

The pattern of denouncement, containment, and, ultimately, punishment taken toward student protesters a decade before was repeated to quell falungong. This response also mirrored similar actions taken against certain qigong masters, discussed in chapter 3. On April 30, 1999, a state warning was issued ordering citizens, especially officials, not to participate in forthcoming demonstrations. Whenever protesters tried to show up in large numbers, they were either turned away or detained and sent back home. There was a delay of several weeks before any additional official actions were taken. Then, on July 22,

1999, a concerted antifalungong campaign unfolded. This highly visible and orchestrated crackdown began with the arrests of over seventy key figures and a ban on all practice. All falungong books, posters, and audiotapes and video CDs were ordered to be destroyed, and neighborhood committees, work units, and other social units were brought in to collect the materials. The *Jiefang Ribao* (Liberation daily) claimed that over 1.55 million copies of such materials were confiscated and destroyed (Agence France Presse). Large-scale book burnings were organized in major cities and the provinces. To counter the wide circulation of materials, the government presses quickly published their own texts. On a visit to the People's Press Bookstore in December 1999, a dazzling six-story building with massive columns newly located on Western Changan Avenue, the front doors opened on a revealing sight. To the left of the entrance a large shelf was filled with texts about China's bid to join the World Treaty Organization (WTO). Directly to the right was an equally large bookcase filled with antifalungong and history of cults texts. Nearby a poster with graphic images of victims was prominently displayed. The concurrent framing indicated how intricately linked the eradication of this group was to economic progress.

Immediately after the July 1999 crackdown, on July 22, a FLG experience-sharing conference was held in San Jose, California, at a large downtown hotel. The free event, open to the public, was advertised in local papers as well as on the organization's web site. Before entering the main auditorium, young, muscular male sentries with high-tech wraparound headphones kept watch over everyone entering, though no one was turned away. The majority (at least 95 percent) of the two thousand plus participants were Asian or Asian American. The non-Mandarin speakers and journalists used free headsets for simultaneous English translation. The event was very orchestrated. As each member came to the podium, he or she stood in front of the large ten-foot banner with the FLG insignia and bowed deeply before reading testimony of being healed with falungong. Only one person referred to the events in China. One youthful grandmother, newly arrived from Guilin, started to refer to the tightened controls over followers at home and began to sob. The organizers quickly yanked her offstage to calm her down. After she returned to the stage, she stood by mutely with red eyes as an organizer finished reading her story. At the end of the day, organizers urged members to reflect on the day's events and exhorted them to think about ways to increase membership, especially among non-Chinese friends in America. Free booklets about FLG and copies of Kung's recent lectures in Australia were handed out and quickly grabbed by audience members. The carefully structured event, taking place within thirty-six hours of the first crackdown in China, and the numbers of volunteers were clear evidence of the organizational capabilities of this group. Moreover, the stated intention to involve more Anglo-Americans revealed new directions the FLG movement would soon pursue.

In the ensuing two years (1999–2001), a predictable logic of protest and containment evolved into rituals of popular protest, which Elizabeth J. Perry has described as a "magnetic, mimetic connection between the Chinese state and its would-be challengers" (2001, 176). Both spatial and temporal dimensions of official meaning would be contested by protesters. Whenever a notable date came up, especially on major holidays such as May 1 (International Worker's Day) or October 1 (National Day), falungong protesters would try to evade police blockades to shout slogans and unfurl banners in support of FLG before being briskly surrounded by waiting guards and plainclothes police. Security forces became accustomed to preparing for symbolic protests by lone individuals or small groups of followers during such periods and would step up their watch. By the winter of 1999, the average Beijing citizen could sketch a profile of the typical protester. A gregarious taxi driver explained it in this way, "They look like they are from out of town [waidilaide]. But instead of going to the square to take photos like ordinary tourists, they carry plastic bags or small satchels with their toothbrush and wash cloth, because they know they'll be in the slammer for a while." Between July 22 and October 30, 1999, over 35,000 protesters were detained, including several members holding foreign passports (Pomfret 2002).

The purge of sect members extended far beyond the visible arrests of protesters. All major institutions from party members to the military, media, and other state work units underwent a thorough cleansing of the ranks. During the summer and fall of 1999, each of these entities made public announcements of support for the antifalungong campaign with self-criticisms of former members.[7] Alliances between scientists and medical doctors forged during the early 1990s quickly came back into play.[8] News stories and television broadcasts included stories of how followers died from stopping their medication or suffering a form of psychosis that could lead to violent death. Leading scientists spoke out vehemently, denouncing the group as a cult that promoted superstition (mixin) and disorder, the antithesis of science.

The war against falungong and mixin was waged on several media fronts. Earlier I addressed how significant the Internet was in facilitating communication for many qigong groups. Like faxes and international radio broadcasts during the unrest of 1989, in 1999 the Internet proved to be as complicated for the PRC to contain. When the government announced its ban, several falun web sites quickly posted "eyewitness" accounts of the crackdown. Letters of protest flooded the sites. Even Kung posted a letter stating his public response to the Chinese government's efforts to extradite him back to China. Within a few days, all falun-related web sites operating within the mainland were shut down, while various official government news sources went online with new accounts about the false and superstitious practices falun represented. Access to the Internet for users in China became restricted as many servers were shut down. Even though followers began to rely on alternative forms of communication, the broad presence of falungong on the Internet continued to draw officials' attention to this medium. Subsequently, cybercafés were temporarily closed down, and operators of dissident web sites were arrested.

Television was a key medium where the state expounded its view of the sect as an evil cult. From July 21 to 25, 1999, a government documentary on falungong was repeatedly shown on national television.[9] Regular programming was canceled, and the special presentation aired even as far away as Tibet. Stories of family tragedies—members who committed suicide, participated in violent acts, or died from ceasing medication—took center stage. Sobbing relatives told painful tales of the demise of family members while graphic images were televised. Such narratives served to illustrate how the sect had "disrupted social order" (*pohuai shehui wending*). The video contrasted claims by founder Kung with testimonials of former disciples to proclaim that falungong was not a higher form of knowledge. Toward the end of the documentary, ordinary practitioners who simply sought healing were excused for having been duped by Kung; however, they were urged to undergo serious revamping of their thoughts (*sixiang*). Another state documentary that emerged during this period featured a young, urbane reporter who conducted an interview with the head of the Chinese Academy of Sciences. Dressed neatly in a white shirt and tie, the scientist compared antisuperstition campaigns in the twentieth century. The first took place in 1927 in Hunan to suppress superstition among peasants. All revolutionary workers at the Jiangxi base camp underwent training to combat rural superstitions. From 1949 to 1952, there were three campaigns against mixin. The discussion indicated that the state response toward falungong followed a long history of concern about sectarian activity that could potentially undo socialist reforms and modernization.

The flexible accumulation of FLG followers and influence outside China continues to provoke the leadership at home. In the midst of the nation's expansion and concomitant desire to make China the center of the world once more, falungong has been a thorn in the side of the body politic. The movement embodied social disorder for the state yet gave meaning to those who were being displaced in the new economic order. Individuals who were drawn to the healing and spiritual practices, ordinary men and women in their forties up to their seventies, were the very people who had sacrificed their lives in the forging of the nation. Followers were drawn to the messages of inclusion, especially those who had lost jobs or health care benefits.

In sum, the five-week antifalungong campaign followed a familiar path of declaring heterodox rebellion and establishing legitimacy with strict countermeasures. Despite retractions by Kung, in which he claimed not to be a deity or a reincarnation of Buddha but an "ordinary man" and stated that he was not responsible for organizing the protests, the line had already been crossed. When over 10,000 followers placed themselves in front of Zhongnanhai with additional provocation from an Internet campaign, the Chinese leadership was impelled to save face through strict countermeasures.

MILLENARIAN MOVEMENTS

Many observers have remarked on the similarities of falungong to secret societies and millenarian sects with end of empire messages in China's past. The dramatic confrontation before state compounds and the apocalyptic pronouncements of its leader certainly supported this view. The antifalungong campaign was quite similar to historic responses of various Chinese rulers to rebellions. A comparative view of the Qing government's response to White Lotus rebels in the nineteenth century is instructive. After an unsuccessful attempt in 1813 to take over the imperial palace in the Forbidden City, officials took the following steps, according to Susan Naquin: "In order to quell the 8 Trigrams rebellion, the Ching government undertook both organizational and propaganda measures to counteract rebel claims to legitimacy. In the first place it was necessary for the government to secure the loyalty and assistance of the non-rebel population, particularly the local elites. In the second place, it was important to induce the majority of rebel followers to 'return their allegiance' to the Ching" (1976, 232). As the present-day government further tightened the reins of control, a request for the extradition of Kung was sent to Interpol. Though this was ultimately denied, the battle to present the "truth" to Chinese and international audiences continued to be waged on the Internet.

The crackdown on falungong resonates eerily with responses to sectarian organizations in the recent Chinese past. Most Western media were quick to locate the falun followers within a long history of resistance movements such as the White Lotus rebels, Yellow Turbans, and Boxers. Certainly key elements—the presence of a charismatic leader, effervescent transmission of knowledge via devotees, and mental and physical exercises based on qi—were common to all these groups. What follows is an analysis of the elements or preconditions necessary for the spread of charismatic sects and millenarian organizations. Rather than simply concluding that these groups are essentially different variations of the same movements based on qi, I will argue that several interventions in the late twentieth century reveal distinctions between the falun group and previous organizations.

In his analysis of millenarian movements such as the ghost dance, a revival of Native American unity in the mid-nineteenth century, Anthony F. C. Wallace (1961) noted that charismatic leaders were often at the core of such social movements. The initial conversion or origin of a leader's transformation would often be mythologized and used as a catalyst for the group's progression from small bands of believers to regional and even national organizations with hierarchies of status and power. While the presence, or even the mere projection, of a leader has been viewed as the most crucial element of sectarian politics, I contend that the social conditions that lead to the emergence and appeal of a particular leader offer more insight into the nature of such groups. As historians of China have shown, examining the local conditions that lead to the rise and fall of particular groups illuminates further how certain personages and their messages traveled within networks of belief and obligation. Effervescence, or the rapid spread of an organization and related ideologies, is based on Durkheim's concept that events are experienced quite differently in large numbers. The larger social body or communal setting offers compelling moments, sometimes coercive, when individual can lose themselves in the larger entity. Similar moments of effervescence, when the collective experience or crowd mentality is encouraged, can be seen in evangelical faith healing, rock concerts, and qigong performances. In all these groups, past and present, the often eclectic transformation from local group to larger regional alliance is initially based on transformational experiences that facilitate the conversion process of individuals to align themselves with the larger organization. Techniques such as deep breathing, guided imagery, sleight-of-hand performances, and group healing sessions all further convince individuals to participate.

What distinguished millenarian movements from other spiritual organizations with charismatic leaders was the persistent belief that the existing world order was troubled, corrupt, and doomed to end. Only through avid participation in the social movement, including political action, even at times acts of violence or outright warfare, could one be saved from eventual destruction. For several centuries, China has seen the emergence of numerous millenarian movements that have threatened the legitimacy of existing rule and social stability, such as the Boxers, the broad-based group known as the White Lotus rebels, and the Yiguandao sect. Such sectarian organizations share similar views about the corruption of a particular regime and the need for apocalyptic endings. As David Ownby has pointed out, "The condemnation of the sorry state of contemporary morality is a rhetorical strategy shared by many religious groups" (2001, 78). There is a persistent misconception that millenarian movements only happen at the end of each millennium. In fact, such movements occur whenever there is a shift in worldviews catalyzed by persuasive leaders and their helpers, who convert others to the cause. The continued existence of millenarian groups reflects persistent feelings of exclusion and disengagement with the existing social and political order and a desire to forge ties of solidarity and hierarchies that are almost familial.

When millenarian movements develop into political entities and amass great resources, often in the form of human labor and monetary and social capital, it is not surprising that such challenges to existing rule eventually lead to struggles for representation and survival. Mary Douglas, the social anthropologist known best for her analyses of structures and institutions, neatly captures the nearly identical tasks necessary for any entity, whether it is an imperial ruler, socialist bureaucracy, or sectarian organization, to establish and maintain authority.

> Any institution that is going to keep its shape needs to gain legitimacy by distinctive grounding in nature and reason: then it affords to its members a set of analogues with which to explore the world and with which to justify the naturalness and reasonableness of the instituted rules, and it can keep its identifiable continuing form. Any institution then starts to control the memory of its members; it causes them to forget experiences incompatible with its righteous image, and it brings to their minds events which sustain the view of nature that is complementary to itself. It provides the categories of their thought, sets the terms for self-knowledge and fixes identities. All of this is not enough. It must secure the social edifice by sacralizing the principles of justice.   (1986, 112).

Sect leaders denounced the corruptness of regimes while espousing their own hierarchical utopia as an alternative. The Chinese government in imperial periods inevitably responded with full crackdowns to maintain the sacred principle of social order; usually this involved death for sect leaders and reeducation for followers. The long history of shared struggles between millenarian organizations and the Chinese body politic forms a deep pattern of institutional memory that continues to inform contemporary bureaucrats in their responses to recent challengers. The contemporary campaign to eradicate the influence of falungong within China resonates powerfully with this history.

Even though falungong presented many continuities with past millenarian movements, there were also significant differences in its membership. Most of the pre- and early-twentieth-century rebellions were rural, with peasants as the primary participants. The Boxers and White Lotus rebels among others were overwhelmingly described as young and male with few women participants.[10] In contrast, the majority of qigong practitioners, including falungong, tended to be urban based with more or less equal distribution among male and female practitioners at the initiate level. Most qigong devotees were notably older—retired workers, intellectuals, and cadres—people who were solidly based in the socialist system rather than outsiders. As the modes of transmission in the contemporary moment have shifted from the vernacular and visual to include more textual sources such as autobiographical novels, how-to manuals, and the Internet, membership has shifted to incorporate more literate, educated, and elite audiences that also include cadres and scientists. Finally, the more cosmopolitan travel of masters via circuits of greater China and diaspora communities meant that the political arena of containment at home has been entirely transformed. Using foreign press coverage as an intervention in the Chinese mainland has meant that the state also needed to respond at a broader and more unified level at home and abroad as well.

Regulations imposed by state authorities on all forms of qigong healing also increased as a result of the anticult campaign. During the 1990s, qigong practice in parks continued openly despite the medicalization of qigong deviation and licensing of masters. In the winter of 1998, it was still possible to find many eclectic qigong groups practicing in Beijing parks. In the round up of falungong followers, however, which included sweeps in urban parks across the country, many practitioners of other forms found themselves subject to scrutiny and questioning as well. This has had a great impact on the practice of qigong, and many groups have gone underground. Practitioners quietly practice by themselves at home or retreat to the mountains away from official surveillance. Besides qigong practice, members of other spiritual sects such as Zhonggong have been questioned or detained.[11]

PATHOLOGIZING FALUNGONG

It is critical to document the ways in which stories of pathology are utilized and their effects. Sometimes, as chapters 2 and 3 indicate, such stories and illness experiences can mobilize people to seek out charismatic healers in order to try new forms of healing. From the view of the state, the search for alternatives offered key moments for opportunistic masters who needed to be curtailed. As I showed in chapter 4, the new psychiatric category of qigong psychosis was taken up by state officials to call for the regulation of qigong and its masters. When falungong became prominent, reported psychotic episodes attributed to falungong practice provided the state with a key moment: to call for a hard strike campaign. According to state media, 753 cases of deaths related to falungong were reported in 2001.[12] This number more than doubled a year later to over 1600 deaths attributable to delusions and psychotic reactions stemming from falungong practice (McDonald 2002). Gruesome details of some of the most sensational cases of mental instability leading to violent acts were presented on television and newspapers. Continuous narrations of pathology thus served crucial purposes—to counter FLG claims of healing and thereby erode its base of authority and to further illustrate what a cult (*xie jiao*) could do.

On the eve of the Chinese New Year in 2001, five supposed FLG protesters, including a twelve-year-old child, doused themselves with gasoline and set themselves on fire (Dorgan 2001a, b; Pan 2001). Though guards and police on watch at Tiananmen Square rushed to the scene, all the demonstrators suffered severe second- and third-degree burns. Self-immolation has been described in Buddhist practice as the release of the soul from an impure material world. During the Vietnamese-American war, one of the most arresting images was of a Vietnamese Buddhist monk sitting in lotus position while his body burned. Graphic images of the Tiananmen immolations were televised to audiences inured to daily stories about FLG as an evil cult. Another subsequent immolation and follow-up stories about the child's death polarized viewers. Whereas previously many Beijing residents shook their heads at the stubbornness of FLG followers and quietly sympathized with them for their harsh treatment, the immolations were the last straw. The desperate act of the protesters became subject to deft spinning by both FLG organizers and state representatives. Skeptics and conspiracy theorists believed the event was an elaborately staged event intended to discredit FLG and further prove it was an evil cult (Schechter 2000). The falungong spokespeople based in the United States gave notice that these protesters were not true followers as "the teachings of falungong strictly prohibit any form of killing, including suicide" (Schauble 2001). The immolations returned FLG to international headlines after cat-and-mouse demonstrations on Tiananmen Square had become predictable.

Since the first strike in 1999, the state has sent hundreds of FLG followers to detention camps for reeducation and training (Leicester 2001). The majority of falungong practitioners have been sent to special detention centers rather than psychiatric units. Only when practitioners exhibit severe mental disorders are any sent for psychiatric care. Disturbing reports from the FLG organization, foreign media, and Amnesty International about human rights violations and guard brutality have circulated. On the second anniversary of the crackdown, the falungong organization planned a march on Washington, D.C., to urge American policy makers to exert more pressure on this issue. Rather than waiting to respond to further actions on the third anniversary of falungong's protest, the *Renmin Ribao* (People's daily) devoted a half page to the murder of a nine-year-old child by her mother, a falungong practitioner, who believed her daughter was "possessed by a demon and choked her to death."[13] In addition, two survivors of the Tiananmen immolations, who had been carefully rehabilitated in state hospitals, gave public statements about their deluded beliefs.

State media coverage has intensively portrayed falungong as a bizarre public health threat. Any claims of healing by FLG practitioners have been systematically countered with stories of pathology and acts of unthinkable violence prompted by mental instability. Shifting the language and terrain of contestation from legitimacy to pathology has enhanced the ability of officials to mobilize notions of state order. It would be simple to characterize the surreal showdown between falungong organizers and the state as a contest over orthodox beliefs and religious expression. Such readings, however, overlook the profoundly difficult circumstances that bring individuals to search for healing.

CHAPTER EIGHT

SUFFERING AND HEALING

CHINESE CULTS and the state bureaucracy share a long genealogy, bound by a similar desire to claim authority. Dramatic confrontations have been extensively documented in court records and media over the centuries. Yet the compelling reasons explaining why participants become drawn to sectarian groups or engage in subversive activities are little understood and frequently overlooked. The overwhelming majority of practitioners that I encountered sought alternative forms of healing as a response to their own illness. Medical anthropologists, engaged with the critical examination of disease, have long asserted that stories of mental and bodily suffering are indexical of social dis-ease and dislocation. Throughout this book, I have argued that contemporary qigong healing and self-cultivation practices should be viewed within the larger context of the post-Mao market economy, which was on the fast track to modernization. Such an examination facilitates an understanding of how healing practices are shaped by social and political systems and, in turn, how decisions about healing can transform a body politic. The material life and desires of people living in China have dramatically changed since the implementation of economic reforms during the 1980s. Movement toward a globalized market economy within China has also transformed meanings of time and space. Two decades ago, there were few private markets, restaurants, toy stores, or beauty salons in most urban areas. Now, public and private spaces have been refashioned to meet the needs of a population with different material desires and consumption. With visible changes that extend well into rural regions, new forms of consumption continue to deepen existing inequalities. The shifts in everyday life are intricately linked to a changing state bureaucracy that is also adapting to social changes.

In the twenty-first century, the state bureaucracy faces the main issue of how to retain order and control under market liberalism. Old tensions and concerns about social order remain, while the challenge of providing for a younger and very transformed population has become much more complex. With market expansion, shifts in time and space have made the Shanghai minute faster than ever. New social trends that emphasize increased consumption have facilitated bodily discipline as a self-induced order. Such order falls in line with the crucial socialist state project of civilization. Though spiritual civilization was viewed as part of socialist modernity, this notion has been relegated to the overlapping notion of civility (wenming), by which citizens should conduct themselves as proper subjects. The Office of Spiritual Civilization, for instance, was charged with the task of cleaning up foul language and the unsporting behavior of "hooligans" (Chao 2001). In previous spiritual civilization campaigns, habits such as spitting in public were targeted as the main impediments to national progress. It is not surprising that the unbridled forms of healing promoted by falungong directly confronted the regulatory nature of spiritual civilization promoted by the state. Notions of cultivation practiced in such groups were deeply unsettling to the very existence of the state bureaucracy, disrupting notions of order and progress toward material civilization.

The issue of rightful authority has always been a concern with each succession of leaders. In 1992 the government used upcoming anniversaries of the Chinese Communist Party as opportunities to market popular images of the party as revitalized and hip. Old party songs were refashioned as karaoke and disco tunes and distributed for the consumer market rather than as traditional propaganda to send to work units. This strategy was quite different from the Lei Feng campaign that sought to craft socialist morality through the use of old heroes as examples of citizens who placed the party before their own lives. The less-than-enthusiastic reception of this example among urban citizens made the party seek different strategies. Later approaches sought to reinvent the image of the party and state officials as fit and revitalized leaders rather than old-fashioned.

State regulation of qigong attempted to polarize the practice into controlled divisions, either as sport or scientific activity. Public sites were reclaimed for officially sanctioned activities rather than popular pursuits with no boundaries to continued expansion. Deviance from the two arenas of sport and science was deemed the purview of psychiatry and the mental health field. Ultimately, just as workplaces and time were structured, so, too, leisure activities became shaped into politically correct notions. This distinction between public and private spheres meant that qigong as a private activity became subject to public scrutiny. The containment of qigong to specific boundaries of time, space, and movement by the state was antithetical to the very notion of the practice. Qigong inherently was about movement and imagery—movement not only of the body but also of the mind in envisioning the energy of the body. Practitioners sought to release the physical body to cosmological notions of order and time rather than state-imposed order. The connection to trees in qigong practice articulates much more than a turn to the environment in the urban setting. Thousand-year-old gingko, juniper, and cypress trees inside parks are the embodiment of energy, regeneration, and longevity, outlasting most dynasties and political storms. The stories of healing have ensured that I will never view trees, whether southern Louisiana oaks or northern California redwoods, in quite the same way anymore. What is breathtaking about qigong is the stubborn desire to heal and, in the attempt of doing so, not to succumb to the rhythms of the state and its spatial and temporal orders.

Rather than attending to body practices solely at the level of individual experience and the phenomenology of movement, I have emphasized the aesthetics and politics of such practices as potential sites for social movements. As a cultural phenomenon with both local and transnational dimensions, the fervent medical and political response to qigong practice within China reveals much about the nature of political power and the wide influence that qigong masters held. The popular practice of qigong can also be seen as a resurgence of spiritual practice in contemporary times to counter the growing dissolution of socialist policies of modernization. Health practices such as qigong were individual and social strategies to reintegrate the mind and body and counter the increasing chaos of everyday life. Just as the Chinese state has been engaged in constructing social order over the past century, individuals have also sought order of a different nature through the integration of self-cultivation and healing. Practitioners frequently referred to qigong in terms that went beyond techniques of breathing. It was a new way that offered a coherent means to structure daily life amid concerns about reform and corruption. Qigong and other self-healing practices restored a sense of moral codes and breathing room in everyday life.

Neoliberal institutions promoting market liberalization and global trade offer few alternatives to the time-space compression that Jameson (1991) and Harvey (1985b) have identified as characteristic of late capitalism. Studies of Latin America during the 1980s indicate the turn to pentacostalism as a social practice emerged during periods of intense state violence, repression, and neoliberal reform (Lancaster 1988; Quesada 1994). Ethnographic studies of trauma point out that structures of violence that have a stake in the global market contribute to ongoing poverty and unequal access to health care (Farmer 1992,

1999; Kim et al. 2000; Scheper-Hughes 1992). In the present imaginary of globalization, many anthropologists consider the hegemony of market logic and irrationality as a call to action. Jean and John Comaroff's (1999) analysis of "occult economies" in postcolonial South Africa also urges anthropologists to track new formations in which suffering is predicated. In the face of economic restructuring and deepening disparity, we should remain attentive to how people still manage to shape and experience their worlds. A focus on illness narratives, which relates illness to social and moral worlds, still retains a paradigm of pathology. On the other side of illness, however, lie the journeys and attempts made in search of healing.

Such journeys are not easily made. Rather than viewing qigong or any healing practice as simply liberating, we need to understand how bodily transformations for healing are most often enacted through regimens of self-discipline. Biopower, as Foucault has indicated, offers ways to understand this linkage. I suggested, at the outset, that state formations have the potential to be transformed by bodily practices. This was an attempt to reframe views of the Chinese state in particular as a monolithic or top-heavy structure. I have argued that states of embodiment can have profound impact on the state itself. New social spaces and subjectivities can be generative within both organic and political realms. The long history of breathing and healing techniques should be examined next to the coextensive roots of the Chinese bureaucracy to understand formations of biopower both past and present.

The stories of survivors have much to teach us about healing and the will to transform. I remain inspired by the ways in which people create breathing spaces both within themselves and with others. Such spaces demonstrate a perseverance of human will and spirit, which can shake the foundations of any rational state. At the same time, I urge readers to move beyond liberalist tendencies that frame this subjectivity as the triumph of individual will over the political. Instead, we should consider how healing practices enable both individual and political agendas of discipline to be mutually defined through the body. The politics of healing will continue to be the politics of the nation in the twenty-first century.

GLOSSARY

au cun, kang	peace village, health
ansi	suggestion
baoxiao	insured
bigu	Daoist practice of fasting and meditation
bingfang	asylum
dalei	debate
danwei	work unit
danxin	concerned, worried
dao	also referred to as Tao, translated as "the way"
dashi	great master
dian	insanity
donggong	moving qigong
fangshi	recipe masters, Daoist alchemy consultants, or ritual masters
fengshui	literally, wind and water; geomancy art of placement
fengrenyuan	mental asylum
fengzi	mad person
getihu	entrepreneur

gongnengtong	open perceptions
gongyong	public use
guanxi	networks
guocui	national essence
hexiangzhuang	form of qigong
hukou	registered permanent residence
jia	false, fake
jiangwen	reduce fever
jin	2 jin equal 1 kilogram; 1 jin is approximately 1.1023 pounds
jingong	still form of qigong
jingshen jiankang	mental health
jingshen weisheng	mental hygiene
jingshenke bingyuan	psychiatric institute
jinluo	meridian
kang	battle
kexue	science
kexuede qigong	scientific qigong
kuang	violent
laobaixing	literally translates into "old one hundred surnames"; commonly used to refer to ordinary people
laoshi	teacher
lianqi	learning about qi
linggan	sensitive
liuman	hooligan
liuxing	fashionable
luan	chaos, disorder
luohou	backwardness
minjian	folk
mixin	superstition, aberrant belief

moshu	magician
nanke	medicine specializing in male health
nei	internal
neigong	internal qigong
neixiang	introverted
pianzi	swindler
pohuai shehui wending	disrupt social order
qi	vital energy
qigong	movement of vital energy
qigong chupian	qigong-emerging deviation
qigong piancha	qigong-related deviation
qigong suozhi jingsheng zhangai	qigong-induced mental disorder
re	literally, hot; more commonly translated as fever
shaji geihoukan	"kill chicken, scare monkey," a euphemism for setting an example
shehuizhuyi wenming	socialist civilization
shenjing shuairuo	neurasthenia
shenmi	mysterious, mystical
shifu	term for master frequently used in martial arts circles
shinian dongluan	ten years of chaos
shougong	receive energy
suzhi	qualities of a people or population
taiji	a shortened form of taijiquan, usually referred to as tai chi, the martial art form of exercise that involves visualizing the movement of qi as a large ball of energy
teyigongneng	special psychic abilities
tiancai	natural ability
tianming	mandate of heaven

tiaobing	harmonize illness
tudi	disciple or follower
wai	external
waixin	external information, usually hearing voices
wenhua	culture
wenming	civilization
wotou	coarse cornmeal in a cone shape, common in rural North China
wupo	witch
wuxia xiaosuo	martial art novellas
xie	evil
xungen	"search for roots" literary movement during 1980s and 1990s
yijinjing	muscle-tendon–changing qigong
yinggong	hard qigong
yunqi	fortune
yuzhouyu	universal language, a form of speaking in tongues, which was banned as cult practice and pseudoscientific
zhangai	disorder
zheng	true or real, upright
zhengli	create order, clean up
zifei	self-paid
ziwoanshi	autosuggestion
zouhuo rumo	"leave the path and evil will enter," indigenous notion of qigong possession

NOTES

PREFACE

1. The phrase "May you live in interesting times" is considered to be a curse rather than a blessing.
2. See the discussion of double vision in Haraway 1997.

1. INTRODUCTION

1. *Soul Mountain* (2000), by Gao Xingjian, winner of the 2000 Nobel Prize in Literature, documents the search for meaning and self-healing in rural China through the narrator's journey across the country.
2. Formerly known as the Beijing Institute of Iron and Steel Technology, the campus was later upgraded to a university and renamed the China University of Science and Technology in the 1990s.
3. The 1980s was a time when mainland Chinese went abroad to study. I was constantly asked whether I had connections that could help in sponsoring a friend or their relatives.
4. For instance, the phrase *shendi luogen* refers to overseas Chinese who are the branches or extensions of deeper family roots in local provinces.
5. Gay Becker (1997) also notes this relationship between breath and pathology or wellness in her ethnography on the disruption of illness and disease.
6. When I was a teenage novice in martial arts, instructors would share stories about the incredible abilities of certain masters.
7. Aside from the case of the Taiping Rebellion in the mid–nineteenth century (1840–50), during which transmission of knowledge based on evangelical Chris-

tian conversion spread rapidly among rural villages and sparked a sectarian movement.

8. Barend ter Haar (1998) and David Ownby (1996, 2001) have raised concerns about the term "White Lotus," which was used perjoratively in official records.

9. Later, in chapter 6, I will examine the notion of *mixin*, the indigenous form of beliefs and practices that signify superstition.

10. John O'Neill (1985) discussed numerous functions and five entities of the body (world, social, politic, consumer, and medical) related to power and its reproduction.

11. The health of a national leader is still followed quite closely. For instance, the results of any physical exams of U.S. presidents are often broadcast as world news. Moreover, leaders commonly remark on the need for bodily and dietary regimens for stronger nation-states. For a discussion of how leaders such as Mao and Gandhi embodied national ideals of socialist and postcolonial states, see Li (1994) and Alter (2000).

12. Doreen Massey's reading of Lefebvre in particular has addressed how the spatial organization of society makes much difference in the ways in which the social operates.

13. This theme has been represented in films such as Terry Gilliam's *Brazil* and the Wachovski Brother's *The Matrix*.

14. As Dutton asserts in his analysis of globalization and rights in China, Western liberal accounts of rights further portray the otherness of China and those who exist outside the system (1999, 74).

15. For instance, citations and keyword categories pertaining to complementary and alternative medicines in Medline, a medical research database, increased at an exponential level during the 1990s.

16. As I will address in chapter 4, some of these symptoms were viewed as a routine part of daily practice. In some martial art practices, such sensations were viewed as an indication of successful practice, signaling that the practitioner was ready to progress to the next level of knowledge once the purgative effects of these symptoms concluded.

17. I will discuss further in the next chapter my use of the term "late socialist" rather than "postsocialist" to describe conditions in China.

2. FEVER

1. Train rides, the primary means of long-distance travel across China, offered a microcosm of society. Trains usually had three fares, or classes, of service: hard seat (*yingzuo*), hard sleeper (*yingwo*), and soft sleeper (*ruanwo*). University students traveling home for spring festival often rode in the hard seat section along with others traveling on limited funds. Seats in this section, which easily accommodated over one hundred passengers, were largely unreserved, so boarding was frenzied, passengers throwing their bags and sometimes passing young

children through windows to claim a seat before those squeezing onto the train. In contrast, the soft sleeper compartment had four cushioned mattresses with sheets per closed cabin and was usually reserved for cadres or foreigners. The hard sleeper section had six bunk beds in open sections. As a journey commenced, metal cups and recycled jars filled with tea or instant noodles would be taken out for hot water as train attendants rolled an industrial-size kettle through the aisles. Loud broadcasts of Chinese opera, pop music, or daily news would blare through each train car. Through the din, meal times were moments when strangers together for the journey would exchange small talk or gather special tips on their destinations.

2. The notion of the superorganic was also a key concept in American anthropology during the 1930s.

3. I am grateful to L. Yuan for explaining these to me.

4. See also Barmé (1999) for a discussion of this era.

5. Judith Farquhar (1996) includes a detailed discussion of Lei Feng and the revitalized 1990 campaign.

6. This was a frequent statement during the fifties and sixties, meant to reverse the "sick men of Asia" image. For more on Mao fever, see Barmé and Jaivin (1992).

7. In English, most writing about qigong has been instructional or autobiographical, authored by both Chinese and Euro-American masters. See, e.g., Yang 2000; K. Cohen 1997.

8. In an ironic corollary, a state publishing house has recently printed official translations of the Harry Potter series, which has been wildly popular worldwide during the late 1990s. Though the novels are based on accounts of magical powers and potentially contradict state discouragement of superstition (*mixin*), their publication has been widely supported by the state.

3. RIDING THE TIGER

1. Sun Simiao, a Tang dynasty physician renowned for his healing abilities, was eventually elevated into a popular folk figure known as the medicine king (*yao wang*). He is frequently portrayed with a dragon and tiger, his knee often resting on the tiger (see Unschuld 1986, 88–96).

2. It is important to note that not all newspapers took the same view. More popular dailies such as *Guangming Ribao* and *Beijing Ribao* were sympathetic to Master Xu and continued to publish articles about her abilities. The two papers mentioned in the text are state publications that voice official views.

4. QIGONG DEVIATION OR PSYCHOSIS

1. The wide range of terms describing deviation included, among others, *dantian qigu* (where qi is stuck in the dantian point in the lower abdomen), *lo qi* (losing qi essence), *neiqi buzhi* (internal qi not circulating according to principles), *qi lu-*

anchuan (qi moving chaotically), *sanshi* (literally, "three corpses," referring to the movements that bring on possession: shakes, uncontrollable thoughts, and uncontrollable words), and *taishan yading* (Mount Tai pressing down on the head).

2. See Hahn (1995) about range of meanings of medicalization.
3. According to Sing Lee (personal communication, December 2001), the DSM committee had a much longer list of culture-bound syndromes and categories. Rather than incorporating the expanded version in the text and acknowledging the central role that culture plays in mental health and illness, the DSM-IV only added the information as an appendix.
4. Personal communication.

5. CHINESE PSYCHIATRY AND THE SEARCH FOR ORDER

1. Many university campuses functioned as autonomous work units with their own restaurants, dining halls, markets, post offices, stores, nursery schools, housing blocks, and public showers/baths.
2. Luhrmann (2000) addresses the development of intuition as a professional skill in American psychiatry.
3. Ng notes that *diankuang* cases were widely viewed as yin-yang disturbances (1990, 34). Porkert (1974, 227) also discusses kuang.
4. Such strategies continue to be employed by desperate family members in modern society. During a visit to Taiwan in 1992, psychiatric professionals related to me how relatives who were mentally ill or suffering from Alzheimer's disease would be driven to remote rural areas and abandoned.
5. China Medical Board Inc., box 96, folder 689, Rockefeller Foundation Archives.
6. China Medical Board Series II, letter from A. M. Dunlap to R. S. Greene, box 53, folder 1239, Rockefeller Foundation Archives.
7. China Medical Board, February 6, 1923, box 96, folder 689, Rockefeller Foundation Archives.
8. This figure was derived from comparative data in Japan. There was a ratio of one mad person to every four hundred people in Japan at the time. China Medical Board Inc., box 96, folder 689, Rockefeller Foundation Archives.
9. China Medical Board Inc., box 66, folder 467, Rockefeller Foundation Archives.
10. China Medical Board Inc. box 22, folder 155, Rockefeller Foundation Archives.
11. Robin Munro's examination of Chinese forensic or judicial psychiatry notes that special *ankang* (peace and health) facilities for the criminally insane were established in 1987 (2000). He also acknowledges that general psychiatry operates as a distinct entity from the specialization in forensics.

6. MANDATE OF SCIENCE

1. Acknowledging Stanley Tambiah's (1990) intellectual history of the science of anthropology, Laura Nader's introduction to *Naked Science* (1996) contextualizes

the formations of science relative to debates about magic and science that anthropologists such as Tylor, Fraser, and Malinowski addressed in the late nineteenth and early twentieth centuries. The work of Malinowski especially acknowledged indigenous knowledge, which remains a prominent research direction for comparative studies of science.

2. The circumstances of his return are discussed extensively by Iris Chang (1995) as well as on several web sites, the most notable being the Federation of American Scientists.'

3. 1999 International Yan Xin Qigong Association, http://www.twm.co.nz/sai/DrYan_qi.htm, June 11, 2001; emphasis in the original.

4. Francesca Bray's (1997) reading of Needham's work offers a compelling assessment of its consequences.

5. See Spence (1984) and Waley-Cohen (1999) for further discussion of this site in historical context.

6. The May Fourth Movement, following protests of the Versailles Treaty of 1919, coalesced into fervent social, literary, and political activity that questioned Chinese culture and China's place in the modern world. The rejection of the traditional principles of Confucianism and patriarchy, for instance, opened up new intellectual directions that embraced science as well as Western art and culture.

7. TRANSNATIONAL QIGONG

1. Jeffrey Meyer (1991) has a wonderful discussion of sacred space and the layout of Beijing. For a discussion of the floating population, see Dorothy Solinger (1999).

2. The Third World Congress on Qigong took place in the fall of 1999, again in San Francisco.

3. Manuel Castells (1996) has described network society to be one in which new forms of information flow and circulate to facilitate the production not only of goods but of selves.

4. As with other masters in this book, I will refer to this person by pseudonym.

5. Zibin Guo (1999) provides an excellent discussion of the different generations, linguistic communities, and classes in the Chinese American and immigrant community.

6. Such a move can be traced back even to the mid-Qing era in which "it was very common for sects to find themselves in competition with each other for followers" (Gaustad 2000, 4).

7. "Persist in Strict Management of the Party," *Renmin Ribao* (People's daily), July 26, 1999.

8. "Fight Against Pseudoscience Important," *China Daily* (*Zhongguo Ribao*), July 26, 1999.

9. I am grateful to Anthony Kuhn, who sent a copy of this video.

10. Historians of Chinese sectarian movements and rebellions have noted that many different groups were often lumped together or characterized as "White Lotus" or

"Boxers" despite distinctly different self-identification among groups. See Haar 1998 and Gaustad 2000.

11. " 'National-Gong' Sect Leader Arrested in Sichuan," Agence France Presse, November 1, 1999.

12. "Over 700 Falungong Practitioners Die Unjustly," *Renmin Ribao* (People's daily), August 9, 1999.

13. Ibid.

BIBLIOGRAPHY

Agnew, James and John Duncan, eds. *The Power of Place: Bringing Together Geographical and Sociological Imaginations*. Boston: Unwin Hyman, 1989.

Alter, Joseph S. *Gandhi's Body: Sex, Diet, and the Politics of Nationalism*. Philadelphia: University of Pennsylvania Press, 2000.

Altorki, Soraya and Camillia Fawzi El-Solh, eds. *Arab Women in the Field: Studying Your Own Society*. Syracuse, N.Y.: Syracuse University Press, 1988.

Altshuler, L. L., X. D. Wang, H. Q. Qi, Q. A. Hua, W. W. Q. Wang, and M. L. Xia. "Who Seeks Mental Health Care in China? Diagnoses of Chinese Outpatients According to DSM-III Criteria and the Chinese Classification System." *American Journal of Psychiatry* 145, no. 7 (1988): 872–75.

Anagnost, Ann. *National Past-Times: Narrative, Representation, and Power in Modern China*. Durham, N.C.: Duke University Press, 1997.

Anderson, Benedict. *Imagined Communities: Reflections on the Origins and Spread of Nationalism*. London: Verso, 1983.

——. *Language and Power: Exploring Political Cultures in Indonesia*. Ithaca: Cornell University Press, 1990.

Ao, Fu. "Ruci Liangong" (How to practice qigong). *Zhongguo Tiyubao* (Chinese sports news), April 1, 1990.

Appadurai, Arjun. *The Social Life of Things: Commodities in Cultural Perspective*. Cambridge: Cambridge University Press, 1986.

——. *Modernity at Large: Cultural Dimensions of Globalization*. Minneapolis: University of Minnesota Press, 1996.

Armstrong, David. *The Political Anatomy of the Body*. Cambridge: Cambridge University Press, 1987.

Babaian, E. A. (Eduard Armenakovich), with Yu. G. Shashina. *The Structure of Psychiatry in the Soviet Union.* Trans. Vladimir N. Brobov and Boris Meerovich. New York: International Universities Press, 1985.

Bachelard, Gaston. *The New Scientific Spirit.* Trans. Arthur Goldhammer. Boston: Beacon, 1984.

Bachelard, Gaston. *The Poetics of Space.* Trans. Maria Jolas. Boston: Beacon, 1994.

Balsamo, Anne. *Technologies of the Gendered Body: Reading Cyborg Women.* Durham, N.C.: Duke University Press, 1996.

Barlow, Tani. ed. *Gender Politics in Modern China: Writing and Feminism.* Durham, N.C.: Duke University Press, 1993.

——. "Theorizing Woman: Funu, Guojia, Jiating (Chinese Woman, Chinese State, Chinese Family)." In *Body, Subject, and Power in China,* ed. Angela Zito and Tani E. Barlow, 253–89. Chicago: University of Chicago Press, 1994.

Barmé, Geremie R. *Shades of Mao: The Posthumous Cult of the Great Leader.* Armonk, N.Y.: Sharpe, 1996.

——. *In the Red: On Contemporary Chinese Culture.* New York: Columbia University Press, 1999.

Barmé, Geremie and Linda Jaivin, eds. *New Ghosts, Old Dreams: Chinese Rebel Voices.* New York: Times Books, 1992.

Barmé, Geremie and John Minford, eds. *Seeds of Fire.* New York: Hill and Wang, 1988.

Barrett, Robert. "Clinical Writing and the Documentary Construction of Schizophrenia." *Culture, Medicine, and Psychiatry* 12, no. 3 (1988): 265–300.

Bartlett, Annie. "Spatial Order and Psychiatric Disorder." In *Architecture and Order: Approaches to Social Space,* ed. Michael Parker Pearson and Colin Richards. London: Routledge, 1994.

Basaglia, Franco. "Madness/Delirium." In *Psychiatry Inside Out: Selected Writings of Franco Basaglia,* ed. Nancy Scheper-Hughes and Anne M. Lovell. New York: Columbia University Press, 1987.

Bataille, Georges. *Inner Experience.* Trans. Leslie Anne Boldt. Albany: SUNY Press, 1988.

Becker, Gaylene. *Disrupted Lives: How People Create Meaning in a Chaotic World.* Berkeley: University of California Press, 1997.

Becker, Robert O. and Gary Selden. *The Body Electric: Electromagnetism and the Foundation of Life.* New York: Morrow, 1985.

Benson, Herbert. *The Mind/Body Effect: How Behavioral Medicine Can Show You the Way to Better Health.* New York: Simon and Schuster, 1979.

——. *Beyond the Relaxation Response: How to Harness the Healing Power of Your Personal Beliefs.* New York: Times Books, 1984.

Berrios, German E. and Roy Porter, eds. *A History of Clinical Psychiatry: The Origin and History of Psychiatric Disorders.* New York: New York University Press, 1995.

Birnbaum, Raoul. *The Healing Buddha.* Rev. ed. Boston: Shambhala, 1989.

Blecher, Marc J. *China, Politics, Economics, and Society: Iconoclasm and Innovation in a*

Revolutionary Socialist Country. Marxist Regime Series. London: F. Pinter; Boulder, Colo.: L. Reinner, 1986.

Blunt, Alison and Gillian Rose, eds. *Writing Women and Space: Colonial and Postcolonial Geographies*. New York: Guilford, 1994.

Bloch, Sidney and Paul Chodoff. *Psychiatric ethics*. 2d ed. Oxford: Oxford University Press, 1991.

Bloch, Sidney and Peter Reddaway. *Soviet Psychiatric Abuse: The Shadow Over World Psychiatry*. London: Gollancz, 1984.

Bloom, Gerald. "Primary Health Care Meets the Market in China and Vietnam." *Health Policy* 44, no. 3 (June 1998): 233–52.

Bloom, G. and X. Y. Gu. "Health Sector Reform: Lessons from China." *Social Science and Medicine* 45, no. 3 (August 1997): 351–60.

Bloom, G. and D. McIntyre. "Towards Equity in Health in an Unequal Society." *Social Science and Medicine* 47, no. 10 (November 1998): 1529–38.

Bloom, G. and T. Shenglan. "Rural Health Prepayment Schemes in China: Towards a More Active Role for Government." *Social Science and Medicine* 48, no. 7 (April 1999): 951–60.

Bodde, Derk. *Chinese Thought, Society, and Science: The Intellectual and Social Background of Science and Technology in Pre-modern China*. Honolulu: University of Hawaii Press, 1991.

Bond, Michael, ed. *The Psychology of the Chinese People*. Hong Kong: Oxford University Press, 1986.

Bosco, Joseph. "Yiguan Dao: 'Heterodoxy' and Popular Religion in Taiwan." In *The Other Taiwan: 1945 to the Present*, ed. Murray A. Rubinstein, 423–44. Armonk, N.Y.: Sharpe, 1994.

Bourdieu, Pierre. *Outline of a Theory of Practice*. Trans. Richard Nice. Cambridge: Cambridge University Press, 1977.

———. *Distinction: A Social Critique of the Judgement of Taste*. Cambridge: Harvard University Press, 1984.

Bourguignon, Erika, ed. *Religion, Altered States of Consciousness, and Social Change*. Columbus: Ohio State University Press, 1973.

Bowker, Geoffrey C. and Susan Leigh Star. *Sorting Things Out: Classification and Its Consequences*. Cambridge, Mass.: MIT Press, 1999.

Bray, Francesca. *Technology and Gender: Fabrics of Power in Late Imperial China*. Berkeley: University of California Press, 1997.

Bredon, Juliet. *Peking: A Historical and Intimate Description of Its Chief Places of Interest*. London: T. Werner Laurie, 1924.

Brownell, Susan. *Training the Body for China: Sports in the Moral Order of the People's Republic*. Chicago: University of Chicago Press, 1995.

Brownell, Susan and Jeffrey N. Wasserstrom, eds. *Chinese Femininities/Chinese Masculinities: A Reader*. Foreword Thomas Laqueur. Berkeley: University of California Press, 2002.

Buck Morss, Susan. *The Dialectics of Seeing: Walter Benjamin and the Arcades Project.* Cambridge, Mass.: MIT Press, 1989.

Bulgakov, Mikhail. *The Master and Margarita.* Trans. Mirra Ginsberg. New York: Grove, 1967.

Bullock, Mary Brown. *An American Transplant: The Rockefeller Foundation and Peking Union Medical College.* Berkeley: University of California Press, 1980.

Burridge, Kenelm. *Mambu: A Melanesian Millennium.* Princeton: Princeton University Press, 1995.

Butler, Judith P. *The Psychic Life of Power: Theories in Subjection.* Stanford, Calif.: Stanford University Press, 1997.

Bynum, W. F., Stephen Lock, and Roy Porter. *Medical Journals and Medical Knowledge: Historical Essays.* London: Routledge, 1992.

Bynum, W. F. and Roy Porter, eds. *Medical Fringe and Medical Orthodoxy, 1750–1850.* London: Croom Helm, 1987.

Bynum, W. F., Roy Porter, and Michael Shepherd, eds. *The Anatomy of Madness: Essays in the History of Psychiatry.* Vol. 1, *People and Ideas.* London: Tavistock, 1985a.

——. *The Anatomy of Madness: Essays in the History of Psychiatry.* Vol. 2, *Institutions and Society.* London: Tavistock, 1985b.

Calloway, Paul. *Russian/Soviet and Western Psychiatry: A Contemporary Comparative Study.* New York: Wiley, 1993.

Calvino, Italo. *Invisible Cities.* Trans. William Weaver. New York: Harcourt, Brace, 1972.

Canguilhem, Georges. *The Normal and the Pathological.* Cambridge, Mass.: MIT Press, 1989.

Cannon, Walter B. *The Wisdom of the Body.* New York: Norton, 1939.

Cao, Zhonghua. "Yan Xin Shaozuo Xiedaogong Baogao Weituo" (Yan Xin should give lessons without carrying on the qigong). *Zhongguo Tiyubao* (Chinese exercise news), April 8, 1990.

Carrin, G., A. Ron, H. Yang, H. Wang, et al. "The Reform of the Rural Cooperative medical System in the People's Republic of China: Interim Experience in 14 Pilot Counties." *Social Science and Medicine* 48, no. 7 (April 1999): 961–72.

Castel, Robert. *The Regulation of Madness: The Origins of Incarceration in France.* Trans. W. D. Halles. Berkeley: University of California Press, 1988.

Castel, Robert, F. Castel, and Anne Lovell. *The Psychiatric Society.* New York: Columbia University Press, 1981.

Castells, Manuel. *The City and the Grassroots: A Cross-Cultural Theory of Urban Social Movements.* London: Edward Arnold, 1983.

——. *The Rise of the Network Society.* Cambridge, Mass. Blackwell, 1996.

——. *End of Millennium.* Malden, Mass.: Blackwell, 1998.

Certeau, Michel de. *The Practice of Everyday Life.* Trans. Steven Rendall. Berkeley: University of California Press, 1984.

Chan, Anita, Richard Madsen, and Jonathan Unger. *Chen Village Under Mao and Deng.* Rev. ed. Berkeley: University of California Press, 1992.

Chang, Iris. *Thread of the Silkworm*. New York: Basic, 1995.

Chao, Julie, "Beware the Beijing Curse." *South China Morning Post*, June 15, 2001.

Chen, C. C. *Medicine in Rural China*. Berkeley: University of California Press, 1988.

Chen, Nancy N. "Urban Spaces and Experiences of *Qigong*." In *Urban Spaces in Contemporary China*, ed. Deborah Davis, Richard Kraus, Barry Naughton, and Elizabeth Perry, 347–61. Cambridge: Woodrow Wilson Center Press and Cambridge University Press, 1995.

———. "Translating Psychiatry and Mental Health in Twentieth-Century China." In *Tokens of Exchange: Problems of Translation in Global Circulation*, ed. Lydia Liu, 305–27. Durham, N.C.: Duke University Press, 1999.

———. "Cultivating Qi and the Body Politic." *Harvard Asia Pacific Review* 4, no 1 (winter 2000): 45–49.

———. "Health, Wealth, and the Good Life in Contemporary China." In *Ethnographies of the Urban in Late Twentieth Century China*, ed. Nancy N. Chen, Constance Clark, Suzanne Gottschang, and Lyn Jeffery, 165–82. Durham, N.C.: Duke University Press, 2001.

———. "Embodying Qi and Masculinities in Post Mao China." In *Chinese Femininities/Chinese Masculinities: A Reader*, ed. Jeffrey N. Wasserstrom and Susan Brownell, 315–29. Berkeley: University of California Press, 2002.

Cheseneaux, Jean, ed. *Popular Movements and Secret Societies in China, 1840–1950*. Stanford, Calif.: Stanford University Press, 1972.

Cheung, F. M. "Conceptualization of Psychiatric Illness and Help-seeking Behavior Among Chinese." *Culture, Medicine, and Psychiatry* 11, no. 1 (1987): 97–106.

Chin, Robert S. and Ai-Li S. Chin. *Psychological Research in Communist China, 1949–1966*. Cambridge, Mass.: MIT Press, 1987.

China Medical Board Papers. Rockefeller Foundation Archives, Rockefeller Archive Center, North Tarrytown, New York.

Chinese Medical Association. *Chinese Classification of Mental Disorders*. 2d ed. Hunan: Hunan Medical University, 1989.

———. *Chinese Classification of Mental Disorders*. 3d ed. Shandong: Shandong Science Technology Press.

Chinese Medical Association and Nanjing Medical University. *Chinese Classification of Mental Disorders*. 2d ed., rev. (CCMD-2-R). Nanjing: Dong Nan University Press.

Chodorow, Nancy. *The Power of Feelings: Personal Meaning in Psychoanalysis, Gender, and Culture*. New Haven, Conn.: Yale University Press, 1999.

Cochrane, Glynn. *Big Men and Cargo Cults*. Oxford: Oxford University Press, Clarendon, 1970.

Cohen, Kenneth S. *The Way of Qigong: The Art and Science of Chinese Energy Healing*. New York: Ballantine, 1997.

Cohen, Lawrence. *No Aging in India: Alzheimer's, the Bad Family, and Other Modern Things*. Berkeley: University of California Press, 1998.

Cohen, Paul A. *History in Three Keys: The Boxers as Event, Experience, and Myth*. New York: Columbia University Press, 1997.

Cohen, Stanley and Andrew Scull. *Social Control and the State*. New York: St. Martin's, 1983.

Comaroff, Jean. *Bodies of Power, Spirits of Resistance*. Chicago: University of Chicago Press, 1985.

Comaroff, Jean and John Comaroff. "Occult Economies and the Violence of Abstraction: Notes from the South African Postcolony." *American Ethnologist* 26, no. 2 (1999): 279–303.

Comaroff, John and Jean Comaroff. *Of Revelation and Revolution: Christianity, Colonialism, and Consciousness in South Africa*. Vol. 1. Chicago: University of Chicago Press, 1991.

———. *Ethnography and the Historical Imagination*. Boulder, Colo.: Westview, 1992.

Conrad, Peter and J. W. Schneider. *Deviance and Medicalization: From Badness to Sickness*. St. Louis: Mosby, 1980.

Csordas, Thomas J. *The Sacred Self: A Cultural Phenomenology of Charismatic Healing*. Berkeley: University of California Press, 1994a.

———. *Language, Charisma, and Creativity: The Ritual Life of a Religious Movement*. Berkeley: University of California Press, 1997.

———, ed. *Embodiment and Experience: The Existential Ground of Culture and Self*. Cambridge: Cambridge University Press, 1994b.

Cui, Yueli. *Public Health in the People's Republic of China*. Beijing: People's Medical Publishing House; Hong Kong: Medical China Publishing, 1986.

Davis, Deborah. *Long Lives: Chinese Elderly and the Communist Revolution*. Rev. ed. Stanford, Calif.: Stanford University Press, 1991.

Davis, Deborah and Steve Harrell, eds. *Chinese Families in the Post-Mao Era*. Berkeley: University of California Press, 1993.

Davis, Deborah, Richard Kraus, Barry Naughton, and Elizabeth Perry, eds. *Urban Spaces in Contemporary China: The Potential for Autonomy and Community in Post-Mao China*. Washington, D.C.: Woodrow Wilson Center and Cambridge University Press, 1995.

Davis, Edward L. *Society and the Supernatural in Song China*. Honolulu: University of Hawaii Press, 2002.

Davis, Winston. *Dojo: Magic and Exorcism in Modern Japan*. Stanford, Calif.: Stanford University Press, 1980.

Dean, Kenneth. *Taoist Ritual and Popular Cults of Southeast China*. Princeton: Princeton University Press, 1993.

———. *Lord of the Three in One: The Spread of a Cult in Southeast China*. Princeton: Princeton University Press, 1998.

Desjarlais, Robert. *Body and Emotion: The Aesthetics of Illness and Healing in the Nepal Himalayas*. Philadelphia: University of Pennsylvania Press, 1992.

Diagnostic and Statistical Manual of Mental Disorders: DSM-IV. 4th ed. Washington, D.C.: American Psychiatric Association, 1994.

Diamant, Neil. "China's Great Confinement? Missionaries, Municipal Elites, and Police in the Establishment of Chinese Mental Hospitals." *Republican China* 19, no. 1 (November 1993): 3–50.

Dirlik, Arif. *After the Revolution: Waking to Global Capitalism*. Hanover, N.H.: University Press of New England, 1994.

Dirlik, Arif, Paul Healy, and Nick Knight, eds. *Critical Perspectives on Mao Zedong's Thought*. Atlantic Highlands, N.J.: Humanities, 1997.

Dong, Paul and Thomas E. Raffill. *China's Super Psychics*. New York: Marlowe, 1997.

Dorgan, Michael. "Five Falun Gong Followers Set Themselves Ablaze in Beijing." Knight Ridder/Tribune News Service, January 24, 2001.

——. "Another Falun Gong Follower Dies by Self-Immolation in Beijing." Knight Ridder/Tribune News Service, February 17, 2001

Douglas, Mary. *Purity and Danger: An Analysis of the Concepts of Pollution and Taboo*. London: Routledge, 1966.

——. *Natural Symbols: Explorations in Cosmology*. New York: Vintage, 1970.

——. *How Institutions Think*. Syracuse, N.Y.: Syracuse University Press, 1986.

Du, Xinke. "Tiantan Gongyuan Lide Gushi" (The story inside Tiantan Park). *Zhongguo Tiyubao* (Chinese exercise news), July 8, 1990.

Duara, Prasenjit. *Culture, Power, and the State: Rural North China, 1900–1942*. Stanford, Calif.: Stanford University Press, 1988.

——. "Knowledge and Power in the Discourse of Modernity—The Campaigns Against Popular Religion in Early Twentieth-Century China." *Journal of Asian Studies* 50, no. 1 (February 1991): 67–83.

——. *Rescuing History from the Nation: Questioning Narratives of Modern China*. Chicago: University of Chicago Press, 1995.

Duncan, Nancy. *BodySpace: Destabilizing Geographies of Body and Gender*. London: Routledge, 1996.

Durkheim, Emile. *Durkheim on Politics and the State*. Ed. Anthony Giddens. Trans. W. D. Halls. Stanford, Calif.: Stanford University Press, 1986.

——. *The Elementary Forms of Religious Life*. Trans. Karen E. Fields. New York: Free, 1995.

Dutton, Michael. *Policing and Punishment in China: From Patriarchy to "The People."* Cambridge: Cambridge University Press, 1992.

——. *Streetlife China*. Cambridge: Cambridge University Press, 1998.

——. "Street Scenes of Subalternity: China, Globalization, and Rights." *Societal Text* 17, no. 3 (1999): 63–86.

Dwyer, Michael. "Rural Poor Suffer Without Mao's Barefoot Medics." *Australian Financial Review*, August 12, 2001.

Eisenberg, David and Thomas Lee Wright. *Encounters with Qi*. London: Cape, 1985.

Eliade, Mircea. *Shamanism: Archaic Techniques of Ecstasy*. New York: Pantheon, 1964.

Ellin, Nan. *Postmodern Urbanism*. 1996. Reprint, Princeton: Princeton Architectural Press, 1999.

Elliott, Alan J. A. *Chinese Spirit-Medium Cults in Singapore*. London: Athlone, 1990.

Elvin, Mark. "Tales of Shen and Xin: Body-Person and Heart-Mind in China During the Last 150 Years." In *Fragments for a History of the Human Body*, ed. Michel Feher, Ramona Naddaff, and Nadia Tazi, part 2, 266–349. Cambridge, Mass.: MIT Press, 1988.

Elvin, Mark and G. W. Skinner. *The Chinese City Between Two Worlds*. Stanford, Calif.: Stanford University Press, 1974.

Englehardt, Ute. "Qi for Longevity in the Tang." In *Taoist Meditation and Longevity Techniques*, ed. Livia Kohn, 263–96. Ann Arbor: Center for Chinese Studies, University of Michigan, 1989.

Esherick, Joseph W. *The Origins of the Boxer Uprising*. Berkeley: University of California Press, 1987.

Estroff, Sue. *Making It Crazy: An Ethnography of Psychiatric Clients in an American Community*. Berkeley: University of California Press, 1981.

Evans-Pritchard, E. E. *Witchcraft, Oracles, and Magic Among the Azande*. Oxford: Oxford University Press.

Fadiman, Anne. *The Spirit Catches You and You Fall Down: A Hmong Child, Her American Doctors, and the Collision of Two Cultures*. New York: Farrar, Straus, 1997.

Fang, Lizhi. *Bringing Down the Great Wall: Writings on Science, Culture, and Democracy in China*. Ed. and trans. James H. Williams. New York: Knopf, 1991.

Farmer, Paul. *AIDS and Accusation: Haiti and the Geography of Blame*. Berkeley: University of California Press, 1992.

——. *Infections and Inequalities: The Modern Plagues*. Berkeley: University of California Press, 1999.

Farquhar, Judith. *Knowing Practice: The Clinical Encounter of Chinese Medicine*. Boulder, Colo.: Westview, 1994.

——. "Market Magic: Getting Rich and Getting Personal in Medicine After Mao." *American Ethnologist* 23, no. 2 (1996): 239–57.

——. "Technologies of Everyday Life: The Economy of Impotence in Reform China." *Cultural Anthropology* 14, no. 2 (May 1999): 155–79.

Featherstone, Mike, Mike Hepworth, and Bryan S. Turner, eds. *The Body: Social Process and Cultural Theory*. London: Sage, 1991.

Fei, Hsiao Tung (Xiao Tung). *Peasant Life in China: A Field Study of Country Life in the Yangtze Valley*. London: Routledge, 1939.

Feng, X. S., S. G. Tang, G. Bloom, M. Segall, et al. "Cooperative Medical Schemes in Contemporary Rural China." *Social Science and Medicine* 41, no. 8 (October 1995): 1111–18.

Feurtado, Gardel MacArthur. *Mao Tse-tung and the Politics of Science in Communist China, 1949–1965*. Ph.D. diss., Stanford University, 1986.

Feld, Steve and Keith Basso, eds. *Senses of Place*. Santa Fe, N.M.: School of American Research Press, 1996.

Feuchtwang, Stephan. *Popular Religion in China: The Imperial Metaphor*. Richmond, Va.: Curzon, 2001.

Feuchtwang, Stephan and Wang Mingming. *Grassroots Charisma: Four Local Leaders in China*. London: Routledge, 2001.

"Fight Against Pseudoscience Important." *China Daily*, July 26, 1999.

Fishbein, Morris. *The New Medical Follies*. New York: Boni and Liveright, 1927.

Foucault, Michel. *The Order of Things*. London: Tavistock, 1970.

——. *Madness and Civilization: A History of Insanity in the Age of Reason*. Trans. Richard Howard. New York: Vintage, 1973.

——. *Discipline and Punish: The Birth of the Prison*. Trans. Alan Sheridan. New York: Vintage, 1979.

——. *The History of Sexuality*. Vol. 1, *An Introduction*. Trans. Robert Hurley. New York: Vintage, 1980a.

——. *Power/Knowledge*. Trans. Colin Gordon. New York: Pantheon, 1980b.

——. *The History of Sexuality*. Vol. 3, *The Care of the Self*. Trans. Robert Hurley. New York: Vintage, 1986.

——. *Mental Illness and Psychology*. Trans. Alan Sheridan. 1976. Reprint, Berkeley: University of California Press, 1987.

——. "Governmentality." In *The Foucault Effect: Studies in Governmental Rationality*, ed. Graham Burcell, Colin Gordon, and Peter Miller, trans. Colin Gordon. Chicago: University of Chicago Press, 1991.

——. *The Birth of the Clinic: An Archaeology of Medical Perception*. Trans. A. M. Sheridan Smith. New York: Random House, 1994.

Frank, Adam. "American Qi: The Representation and Marketing of the Life Force in the U.S.A." Unpublished paper, 1998.

Frankenburg, Ronald, ed. *Time, Health, and Medicine*. London: Sage, 1992.

Franklin, Sarah. "Science as Culture, Cultures of Science." *Annual Review of Anthropology* 24 (1995): 163–84.

Fuller, Robert C. *Mesmerism and the American Cure of Souls*. Philadelphia: University of Pennsylvania Press, 1982.

Furth, Charlotte. *Ting Wen-chiang: Science and China's New Culture*. Cambridge: Harvard University Press, 1970.

——. "Body, Blood, and Gender: Medical Images of the Female Condition in China." *Chinese Science* 7 (1986): 43–66.

——. *A Flourishing Yin: Gender in China's Medical History, 960–1665*. Berkeley: University of California Press, 1999.

Gabriel, Richard A. *Soviet Military Psychiatry: The Theory and Practice of Coping with Battle Stress*. New York: Greenwood, 1986.

Gaines, Atwood, ed. *Ethnopsychiatry: The Cultural Construction of Professional and Folk Psychiatries*. Albany: SUNY Press, 1992.

Gao, Xingjian. *Soul Mountain*. Trans. Mabel Lee. New York: HarperCollins, 2000.

Garden Administration of Beijing. *Famous Ancient Trees in Beijing*. Beijing: Beijing Publishing House, n.d.

Garrett, Clarke. *Spirit Possession and Popular Religion: From the Camisards to the Shakers*. Baltimore: Johns Hopkins University Press, 1987.

Gaubatz, Piper. *Beyond the Great Wall: Urban Form and Transformation on the Chinese Frontiers*. Stanford, Calif.: Stanford University Press, 1996.

Gaustad, Blaine. "Prophets and Pretenders: Inter-sect Competition in Qianlong China." *Late Imperial China* 21, no. 1 (June 2000): 1–40.

Geertz, Clifford. *The Interpretation of Cultures*. New York: Basic, 1973.

Ghosh, Amitav. *The Calcutta Chromosome: A Novel of Fevers, Delirium, and Discovery*. London: Picador, 1996.

Giddens, Anthony. *Modernity and Self-Identity*. Stanford, Calif.: Stanford University Press, 1991.

Gilman, Sander L. *Seeing the Insane*. Chichester: Wiley, 1982.

——. *Difference and Pathology: Stereotypes of Sexuality, Race, and Madness*. Ithaca: Cornell University Press, 1985.

——. *Disease and Representation: Images of Illness from Madness to AIDS*. Ithaca: Cornell University Press, 1988.

——. *Health and Illness: Images of Difference*. London: Reaktion, 1995a.

——. *Picturing Health and Illness: Images of Identity and Difference*. Baltimore: Johns Hopkins University Press, 1995b.

——, ed. *The Face of Madness: Hugh W. Diamond and the Origin of Psychiatric Photography*. Secaucus, N.J.: Citadel, 1976.

Gilmartin, Christina, Gail Hershatter, Lisa Rofel, and Tyrene White, eds. *Engendering China: Women, Culture, and the State*. Cambridge: Harvard University Press, 1994.

Gijswijt-Hofstra, Marijke and Roy Porter, eds. *Cultures of Psychiatry and Mental Health Care in Postwar Britain and the Netherlands*. Amsterdam: Rodopi, 1998.

Gladney, Dru. *Making Majorities: Constituting the Nation in Japan, Korea, China. Malaysia, Fiji, Turkey, and the United States*. Stanford, Calif.: Stanford University Press, 1988.

Goffman, Erving. *Asylums*. Garden City, N.Y.: Doubleday, Anchor, 1961.

Gold, Thomas B. "After Comradeship: Personal Relations in China Since the Cultural Revolution." *China Quarterly*, no. 104 (December 1985): 657–75.

Goldman, H. H., ed. *Review of General Psychiatry*. 2d ed. Norwalk, Conn.: Appleton and Lange, 1988.

Goldman, Merle, Timothy Cheek, and Carol L. Hamrin, eds. *Chinese Intellectuals and the State: In Search of a New Relationship*. Cambridge: Harvard University Press, 1989.

Gong, Y. L., A. Wilkes, and G. Bloom. "Health Human Resource Development in Rural China." *Health Policy and Planning* 12, no. 4 (December 1997): 320–28.

Good, Byron. *Medicine, Rationality, and Experience: An Anthropological Perspective*. Cambridge: Cambridge University Press, 1995.

Good, Byron, Paul Brodwin, Mary-Jo Good, and Arthur Kleinman. *Pain as Human Experience*. Berkeley: University of California Press, 1992.

Goodman, Francis D., Jeannette H. Henney, and Esther Pressel. *Trance, Healing, and Hallucination: Three Field Studies in Religious Experience*. New York: Wiley, 1974.

Gramsci, Antonio. *Selections from the Prison Notebooks*. New York: International Publishers; London: Lawrence and Wishart, 1971.

Granshaw, Lindsay and Roy Porter, eds. *The Hospital in History*. London: Routledge, 1989.

Grosz, Elizabeth. *Volatile Bodies: Toward a Corporeal Feminism*. Bloomington: Indiana University Press, 1994.

———. *Space, Time, and Perversion: Essays on the Politics of Bodies*. New York: Routledge, 1995.

Guangdong Qigong Kexue Yanjiuhui (Guangdong Scientific Qigong Association), eds. *Qigong Yu Kexue* (Qigong and science). No. 100, July. Guangdong Province: Guangdong Scientific Qigong Association, 1991.

Guattari, Felix. *Molecular Revolution: Psychiatry and Politics*. Trans. Rosemary Sheed. New York: Penguin, 1984.

Gui, Zhenzi. "Xun 'Shi' Ji" (The story of seeking the "master"). *Zhongguo Tiyubao* (Chinese exercise news), April 15, 1990.

Guldin, Gregory E. and Aidan Southall, eds. *Urban Anthropology in China*. Leiden, Netherlands: Brill, 1993.

Guo, Zibin. *Ginseng and Aspirin: Health Care Alternatives for Aging Chinese in New York*. Ithaca: Cornell University Press, 2000.

Gupta, Akhil and James Ferguson, eds. *Culture, Power, Place: Explorations in Critical Anthropology*. Durham, N.C.: Duke University Press, 1997.

Gu, Xy, G. Bloom, S. L. Tang, Y. Y. Zhu, et al. "Financing Health Care in Rural China: Preliminary Report of a Nationwide Study." *Social Science and Medicine* 36, no. 4 (February 1993): 385–91.

Haar, Barend J. ter. *Ritual and Mythology of the Chinese Triads: Creating an Identity*. Leiden, Netherlands: Brill, 1998.

Hacking, Ian. *Rewriting the Soul: Multiple Personality and the Sciences of Memory*. Princeton: Princeton University Press, 1995.

———. *Mad Travelers: Reflections on the Reality of Transient Mental Illnesses*. Charlottesville: University Press of Virginia, 1998.

———. *The Social Construction of What?* Cambridge: Harvard University Press, 1999.

Hahn, Robert A. *Sickness and Healing: An Anthropological Perspective*. New Haven: Yale University Press, 1995.

———, ed., with Kate W. Harris. *Anthropology in Public Health: Bridging Differences in Culture and Society*. New York: Oxford University Press, 1999.

Haine, W. Scott. *The World of the Paris Café: Sociability Among the French Working Class*. Baltimore: Johns Hopkins University Press, 1996.

Hannerz, Ulf. *Exploring the City: Inquiries Toward an Urban Anthropology*. New York: Columbia University Press, 1980.

Haraway, Donna. *Modest-Witness@Second-Millennium.FemaleMan-Meets-OncoMouse: Feminism and Technoscience*. New York: Routledge, 1997.

Harding, Susan Friend. *The Book of Jerry Falwell: Fundamentalist Language and Politics*. Princeton: Princeton University Press, 2000.

Harding, Susan, and Charles Bright. *Statemaking and Social Movements: Essays in History and Theory*. Ann Arbor: University of Michigan Press, 1984.

Harper, Donald John. *Early Chinese Medical Literature: The Mawangdui Medical*

Manuscripts. London: Kegan Paul International, 1998; distributed in U.S. by Columbia University Press.

Harvey, David. *Consciousness and the Urban Experience: Studies in the History and Theory of Capitalist Urbanization*. Baltimore: John Hopkins University Press, 1985a.

———. *The Urbanization of Capital: Studies in the History and Theory of Capitalist Urbanization*. Baltimore: Johns Hopkins University Press, 1985b.

———. *The Condition of Postmodernity*. Cambridge: Blackwell, 1989.

Hayles, N. Katherine. *Chaos and Order: Complex Dynamics in Literature and Science*. Chicago: University of Chicago Press, 1991.

He, F. S. "Occupational Medicine in China." *International Archives of Occupational and Environmental Health* 71, no. 2 (March 1998): 79–84.

Helman, Cecil. "Psyche, Soma, and Society: The Social Construction of Psychosomatic Disorders." *Culture, Medicine, and Psychiatry* 9, no. 1 (1985): 1–26.

———. *Culture, Health, and Illness: An Introduction for Health Professionals*. 3d ed. Oxford: Butterworth-Heinemann, 1994.

Henderson, G. E., J. S. Akin, P. M. Hutchinson, S. G. Jin, et al. "Trends in Health Services Utilization in Eight Provinces in China, 1989–1993." *Social Science Medicine* 47, no. 12 (December 1998): 1957–71.

Henderson, Gail and Myron S. Cohen. *The Chinese Hospital: A Socialist Work Unit*. New Haven: Yale University Press, 1984.

Hertz, Ellen. *The Trading Crowd: An Ethnography of the Shanghai Stock Market*. Cambridge: Cambridge University Press, 1998.

Hesketh, T. and W. X. Zhu. "Health in China: The Healthcare Market." *British Medical Journal* 314, no. 7094 (May 31, 1997): 1616–18.

Hess, David. *Spirits and Scientists*. University Park: Pennsylvania State University Press, 1991.

———. *Science in the New Age*. Madison: University of Wisconsin Press, 1993.

———. *Science Studies: An Advanced Introduction*. New York: New York University Press, 1997.

Hinnells, John R. and Roy Porter, eds. *Religion, Health, and Suffering*. London: Kegan Paul International, 1999.

Ho, L. S. "Market Reforms and China's Health Care System." *Social Science and Medicine* 41, no. 8 (October 1995): 1065–72.

Ho, Peng Yoke. *Li, Qi, and Shu: An Introduction to Science and Civilization in China*. Hong Kong: Hong Kong University Press, 1985.

Holston, James and Arjun Appadurai. "Cities and Citizenship." *Public Culture* 8 (1996): 187–204.

Honig, Emily. *Creating Chinese Ethnicity: Subei People in Shanghai, 1850–1980*. New Haven: Yale University Press, 1992.

Honig, Emily and Gail Hershatter. *Personal Voices: Chinese Women in the 1980s*. Stanford, Calif.: Stanford University Press, 1988.

Howes, David, ed. *The Variety of Sensory Experience: A Sourcebook in the Anthropology of the Senses*. Toronto: University of Toronto Press, 1991.

Hsiao, W. C. "The Chinese Health Care System—Lessons For Other Nations." *Social Science and Medicine* 41, no. 8 (October 1995): 1047–55.

Hsiao, W. C. and Y. Liu. "Economic Reform and Health: Lessons from China." *New England Journal of Medicine*, no. 335 (1996): 430–32.

Hsu, Elisabeth. *The Transmission of Chinese Medicine*. Cambridge; Cambridge University Press, 1999.

——. "Spirit (Shen), Styles of Knowing, and Authority in Contemporary Chinese Medicine." *Culture, Medicine, and Psychiatry* 24, no. 1 (2000): 197–229.

Hsu, Francis. *Under the Ancestor's Shadow*. Stanford, Calif.: Stanford University Press, 1971.

Hsu, Francis L. K. *Religion, Science and Human Crises: A Study of China in Transition and Its Implications for the West*. London: Routledge, 1952.

Hu, Chia. *Peking Today and Yesterday*. Peking: Foreign Languages Press, 1956.

Hua, Shiping. *Scientism and Humanism: Two Cultures in Post-Mao China, 1978–1989*. Albany: SUNY Press, 1995.

Hubei Qigong Kexue Yanjiuhui and Hubei Zhongyi Xueyuan (Hubei Qigong Science Association and Hubei Traditional Chinese Medicine College), eds. *Da Zhong Qigong* (Popular qigong). Nos. 6 and 7. Hubei Province: Hubei Qigong Science Association, 1991.

Huff, Toby E. *The Rise of Early Modern Science: Islam, China, and the West*. Cambridge: Cambridge University Press, 1993.

Hu, T. W., M. Ong, Z. H. Lin, and E. Li. "The Effects of Economic Reform on Health Insurance and the Financial Burden for Urban Workers in China." *Health Economics* 8, no. 4 (June 1999): 309–321.

The ICD-10 Classification of Mental and Behavioural Disorders: Clinical Descriptions and Diagnostic Guidelines. Geneva: World Health Organization, 1992.

Ikels, Charlotte. *The Return of the God of Wealth: The Transition to a Market Economy in Urban China*. Stanford, Calif.: Stanford University Press, 1996.

Ingelby, David, ed. *Critical Psychiatry*. New York: Pantheon, 1980.

Isser, Natalie and Lita Linzer Schwartz. *The History of Conversion and Contemporary Cults*. American University Studies Series 7. New York: Lang, 1988.

Ivy, Marilyn. *Discourses of the Vanishing: Modernity, Phantasm, Japan*. Chicago: University of Chicago Press, 1995.

Jameson, Fredric. *Postmodernism; or, The Cultural Logic of Late Capitalism*. Durham, N.C.: Duke University Press, 1991.

Ji, Yi. *Da Qigong Shi Chushan* (The emergence of the great *qi gong* master). Beijing: Hualing Chubanshe, 1990.

Jiang, Shishu, et al. "Taishang Yiren Shuojiao, Taixia Zhongren Kuxiao" (While a person is talking on the platform, many people below are crying and laughing). *Xinmen Wanbao* (New people evening news), March 7, 1990.

Jing, Jun. *The Temple of Memories: History, Power, and Morality in a Chinese Village*. Stanford, Calif.: Stanford University Press, 1996.

Johnson, Frank. "The Western Concept of Self." In *Culture and Self*, ed. Anthony

J. Marsella, George Devos, and Francis L. K. Hsu, 91–139. London: Tavistock, 1985.

——. "Contributions of Anthropology to Psychology," In *Review of Psychiatry*, ed. H. H. Goldman, 2d ed., 180–94. Norwalk, Conn.: Appleton and Lange, 1988.

Johnson, Frank A. *Dependency and Japanese Socialization: Psychoanalytic and Anthropological Investigations into Amae*. New York: New York University Press, 1993.

Johnson, Mark. *The Body in the Mind: The Bodily Basis of Meaning, Imagination, and Reason*. Chicago: University of Chicago Press, 1987.

Jones, Colin and Roy Porter, eds. *Reassessing Foucault: Power, Medicine, and the Body*. London: Routledge, 1994.

Jordan, David K. and Daniel L. Overmyer. *The Flying Phoenix: Aspects of Chinese Sectarianism in Taiwan*. Princeton: Princeton University Press, 1986.

Kahn, Joseph, "China Quietly Shrinks Classic Welfare State, Leaving People to Pay for Pensions, Health Care." *Wall Street Journal*, January 30, 1998, A10.

Kao, John J. *Three Millennia of Psychiatry*. New York: Institute for Advance Research in Asian Science and Medicine, 1979.

Katz, Richard. *Boiling Energy*. Cambridge: Harvard University Press, 1982.

Ke, Yunlu. *Da Qigong Shi* (Great qigong master). Beijing: Renmin Wenxue Chubanshe (People's literature press), 1990.

Kiev, Ari. *Psychiatry in the Communist World*. New York: Science House, 1968.

Kim, Jim Yong, Joyce Millen, Alec Irwin, and John Gershman, eds. *Dying for Growth: Global Inequality and the Health of the Poor*. Monroe, Maine: Common Courage, 2000.

King, Anthony D., ed. *Re-Presenting the City: Ethnicity, Capital, and Culture in the 21st-Century Metropolis*. New York: New York University Press, 1996.

Kingsolver, Ann E., ed. *More than Class: Studying Power in U.S. Workplaces*. Albany: SUNY Press, 1998.

——. *NAFTA Stories: Fears and Hopes in Mexico and the United States*. Boulder, Colo.: Rienner, 2001.

Kipnis, Andrew B. *Producing Guanxi: Sentiment, Self, and Subculture in a North China Village*. Durham, N.C.: Duke University Press, 1997.

Kleinman, Arthur. *Patients and Healers in the Context of Culture*. Berkeley: University of California Press, 1980.

——. *Social Origins of Distress and Disease: Depression, Neurasthenia, and Pain in Modern China*. New Haven: Yale University Press, 1986.

Kleinman, Arthur and Byron Good, eds. *Culture and Depression: Studies in the Anthropology and Cross-Cultural Psychiatry of Affect and Disorder*. Berkeley: University of California Press, 1985.

Kleinman, Arthur and Joan Kleinman. "The Transformation of Everyday Social Experience: What a Mental and Social Health Perspective Reveals About Chinese Communities Under Global and Local Change." *Culture, Medicine, and Psychiatry* 23, no. 1 (1999): 7–24.

———. "Suffering and Its Professional Transformation—Toward an Ethnography of Interpersonal Experience." *Culture, Medicine, and Psychiatry* 15, no. 3 (1991): 275–301.

———. "How Bodies Remember: Social Memory and Bodily Experience of Criticism, Resistance, and Delegitimization Following China's Cultural Revolution." *New Literary History* 25, no. 3 (summer 1994): 707–23.

———. "The Appeal of Experience—The Dismay of Images—Cultural Appropriations of Suffering in Our Times." *Daedalus* 125, no. 1 (winter 1996): 1–23.

Kleinman, Arthur and Tsung-Yi Lin, eds. *Normal and Abnormal Behavior in Chinese Culture*. Dordrecht, Netherlands: Reidel, 1981.

Kleinman, Arthur and David Mechanic. "Mental Illness and Psychosocial Aspects of Medical Problems in China." In *Normal and Abnormal Behavior in Chinese Culture*, ed. Arthur Kleinman and Tsung-yi Lin, 331–56. Dordrecht, Netherlands: Reidel, 1981.

Kleinman, Arthur, Veena Das, and Margaret Lock. *Social Suffering*. Berkeley: University of California Press, 1997.

Kluckhohn, Clyde, ed. *Culture and Behavior: Collected Essays*. New York: Free. 1962.

Knight, Nick, ed. *Mao Zedong on Dialectical Materialism: Writings on Philosophy, 1937*. Armonk, N.Y.: Sharpe, 1990.

Kohn, Livia. *Taoist Mystical Philosophy: The Scripture of Western Ascension*. Albany: SUNY Press, 1991.

———. *Early Chinese Mysticism: Philosophy and Soteriology in the Taoist Tradition*. Princeton: Princeton University Press, 1992.

———, ed. *Taoist Meditation and Longevity Techniques*. Ann Arbor: Center for Chinese Studies, University of Michigan, 1989.

———, ed., with Yoshinobu Sakade. *The Taoist Experience: An Anthology*. Albany: SUNY Press, 1993.

Kondo, Dorinne. *Crafting Selves*. Berkeley: University of California Press, 1991.

Kong, Rong. *Zouhuo Rumo* (Leave the path and evil enters). Beijing: Zhongguo Yiyao Keji Chubanshe (Chinese medical technology press), 1990.

Kroeber, A. L. *Cultural Anthropology in the Problem of Mental Disorder*. New York: McGraw-Hill, 1934.

Kuhn, Philip A. *Soulstealers*. Cambridge: Harvard University Press, 1990.

Kuhn, Thomas S. *The Structure of Scientific Revolutions*. 2d ed. Chicago: University of Chicago Press, 1970.

Kuriyama, Shigehisa. *The Expressiveness of the Body and the Divergence of Greek and Chinese Medicine*. New York: Zone, 1999.

Kwok, D. W. Y. (Danny Wynn Ye). *Scientism in Chinese Thought, 1900–1950*. New Haven: Yale University Press 1965.

Laing, R. D. *The Divided Self*. Harmondsworth: Penguin, 1965.

Lamson, Herbert D. *Social Pathology in China: A Sourcebook for the Study of Problems of Livelihood, Health, and the Family*. Shanghai: Commercial, 1935.

Lancaster, Roger N. *Thanks to God and the Revolution: Popular Religion and Class Consciousness in the New Nicaragua*. New York: Columbia University Press, 1988.

Langford, Jean. "Medical Mimesis: Healing Signs of a Cosmopolitan 'Quack.'" *American Ethnologist* 26, no. 1 (February 1999): 24-46.

Laozi. *Dao de Jing: The Book of the Way.* Trans. and comm. Moss Roberts. Berkeley: University of California Press, 2001.

Laris, Michael. "Chinese TV Twits a Popular Pastime and Gets an Earful on Its Merits." *Washington Post,* July 13, 1998, A13.

Latour, Bruno. *Science in Action: How to Follow Scientists and Engineers through Society.* Cambridge: Harvard University Press, 1987.

——. *Pandora's Hope: Essays on the Reality of Science Studies.* Cambridge: Harvard University Press, 1998.

Latour, Bruno and Steve Woolgar. *Laboratory Life: The Construction of Scientific Facts.* Intro. Jonas Salk. Princeton: Princeton University Press, 1986.

Lau, Kimberly J. *New Age Capitalism: Making Money East of Eden.* Philadelphia: University of Pennsylvania Press, 2000.

Laughing at the Tao: Debates Among Buddhists and Taoists in Medieval China (Hsiao Tao Lun). Trans. and ann. Livia Kohn. Princeton: Princeton University Press, 1995.

Lebra, William P. *Transcultural Research in Mental Health.* Mental Health Research in Asia and Pacific, 2. Honolulu: East West Center, University of Hawaii, 1972.

Lederer, Edith M. "Minister: 600,000 in China Have AIDS." Associated Press, June 26, 2001.

Lee, Sing. "Cultures in Psychiatric Nosology: The CCMD-2-R and International Classification of Mental Disorders." *Culture, Medicine, and Psychiatry* 20, no. 4 (1996): 421–72.

——. "Diagnosis Postponed: Shenjing Shuairuo and the Transformation of Psychiatry in Post Mao China." *Culture, Medicine, and Psychiatry* 23, no. 3 (1999): 349–80.

——. "Chinese Hypnosis Can Cause Qigong-Induced Mental Disorders." *British Medical Journal* 320, no. 7237 (March 18, 2000): 803.

Lee, S. and A. Kleinman. "Psychiatry in Its Political and Professional Contexts: A Response to Robin Munro." *Journal of the American Academy of Psychiatry and the Law* 30, no. 1 (2002): 120–25.

Lefebvre, Henri. *The Production of Space.* Trans. Donald Nicholson-Smith. 1974. Reprint, Cambridge, Mass.: Blackwell, 1991.

——. *Writings on Cities.* Ed. and trans. Eleonore Kofman and Elizabeth Lebas. Oxford: Blackwell, 1996.

Leicester, John. "China Shows Reporters Forbidden Camp." Associated Press, May 22, 2001.

Leland, John and Carla Power. "Deepak's Instant Karma." *Newsweek,* October 20, 1997, 52–60.

Levi, Jean. "The Body: The Daoist's Coat of Arms." In *Fragments for a History of the Human Body,* ed. Michel Feher, Ramona Naddaff, and Nadia Tazi, part 1, 105–26. Cambridge, Mass.: MIT Press, 1988.

Lewis, Dennis. *The Tao of Natural Breathing: For Health, Well-Being, and Inner Growth.* San Francisco: Mountain Wind, 1997.

Lewis, I. M. *Ecstatic Religion: A Study of Shamanism and Spirit Possession*. 2d ed. London: Routledge, 1989.

——. *Religion in Context: Cults and Charisma*. 2d ed. Cambridge: Cambridge University Press, 1996.

Lewis, M. "Chinese Psychiatry After Mao Zedong." *Psychiatric Annuals* 10, no. 6 (1980): 217–24.

Leys, Simon. *Chinese Shadows*. New York: Viking, 1977.

——. *The Chairman's New Clothes: Mao and the Cultural Revolution*. Trans. Carol Appleyard and Patrick Goode. Rev. ed. London: Allison and Busby, 1981.

——. *The Burning Forest: Essays on Chinese Culture and Politics*. New York: Holt, 1986.

Li, Peicai. *Da Ziran De Hunpo* (The soul of the natural world). Beijing: Changhong Chuban Gongsi (Changhong press), 1989.

Li, Yun. "Qigong Yu Qigongxing Jingshen Zhangai" (Qigong and qigong-related mental illness). *Jiankang Ribao* (Health daily), June 9, 1990.

Li, Zhisui. *The Private Life of Chairman Mao: The Memoirs of Mao's Personal Physician*. Trans. Tai Hung-chao, ed. Anne F. Thurston. New York: Random House, 1994.

Li, Zhixin, Yu Li, Guo Zhengyi, Shen Zhenyu, Zhang Honglin, and Zhang Tongling. *Qigong: Chinese Medicine or Pseudoscience?* Amherst, N.Y.: Prometheus, 1999.

Lifton, Robert Jay, *Destroying the World to Save It: Aum Shinrikyo, Apocalyptic Violence, and the New Global Terrorism*. New York: Holt, 1999.

Lifton, Robert Jay. *Thought Reform and the Psychology of Totalism: A Study of "Brainwashing" in China*. New York: Norton, 1961.

Lian, Xingqian, Lu Wei, and Guan Chunfang, eds. *Beijing Kanbing Zhinan* (Beijing medical consultation guidebook). Beijing: Jingji Kexue Chubanshe (Economic science press), 1989.

Lim, R. F. and K. M. Lin. "Cultural Formulation of Psychiatric Diagnosis—Case No. 03, Psychosis Following Qi-Gong in a Chinese Immigrant." *Culture, Medicine, and Psychiatry* 20, no. 3 (1996): 369–78.

Lin, K. M. "Psychopharmacology in Cross-Cultural Psychiatry." *Mount Sinai Journal of Medicine* 63, nos. 5–6 (October–November 1996): 283–84.

Lin, Tsung-Yi. "Neurasthenia Revisited: Its Place in Modern Psychiatry." *Culture, Medicine, and Psychiatry* 13, no. 2 (1989): 105–30.

Lin, Tsung-Yi and Leon Eisenberg, eds. *Mental Health Planning for One Billion People: A Chinese Perspective*. Vancouver: University of Columbia Press, 1985.

Lindenbaum Shirley and Margaret Lock. *Knowledge, Power, and Practice: The Anthropology of Medicine and Everyday Life*. Berkeley: University of California Press, 1993.

Linger, Daniel T. *Dangerous Encounters: Meanings of Violence in a Brazilian City*. Stanford, Calif.: Stanford University Press, 1992.

——. "The Hegemony of Discontent," *American Ethnologist* 20, no. 1 (February 1993): 3–24.

——. "Has Culture Theory Lost Its Minds?" *Ethnos* 22, no. 3 (September 1994): 284–315.

Linton, Ralph. *Culture and Mental Disorders*. Springfield, Ill.: Thomas, 1956.

Litzinger, Ralph A. *Other Chinas: The Yao and the Politics of National Belonging.* Durham, N.C.: Duke University Press, 2000.

Li, S. X. and M. R. Phillips. "Witch Doctors and Mental Illness in Mainland China— A Preliminary Study." *American Journal of Psychiatry* 147, no. 2 (February 1990): 221–24.

Liu, Guangrong and Wu Jiajun, eds. *Zhongguo Qigong Jingdian: Xian Qinzhi Nanbei Chao Bufen I, II* (Classics of Chinese qigong: Before Qin to Nanbei Dynasty I, II). Beijing: Renmin Tiyu Chubanshe (People's physical training press), 1990a.

——. *Zhongguo Qigong Jingdian: Tangchao Bufen I, II* (Classics of Chinese qigong: Tang Dynasty I, II). Beijing: Renmin Tiyu Chubanshe (People's physical training press), 1990b.

——. *Zhongguo Qigong Jingdian: Songchao Bufen I, II* (Classics of Chinese qigong: Song Dynasty I, II). Beijing: Renmin Tiyu Chubanshe (People's physical training press), 1990c.

——. *Zhongguo Qigong Jingdian: Jinyuanchao Bufen I, II* (Classics of Chinese qigong: Jin and Yuan Dynasty I, II). Beijing: Renmin Tiyu Chubanshe (People's physical training press), 1990d.

——. *Zhongguo Qigong Jingdian: Mingchao Bufen I, II* (Classics of Chinese Qigong: Ming Dynasty I, II). Beijing: Renmin Tiyu Chubanshe (People's physical training press), 1990e.

——. *Zhongguo Qigong Jingdian: Qingchao Bufen* (Classics of Chinese qigong: Qing Dynasty). Beijing: Renmin Tiyu Chubanshe (People's physical training press), 1990f.

Liu, Hong and Paul Perry. *Mastering Miracles: The Healing Art of Qi Gong as Taught by a Master.* New York: Warner, 1997.

Liu, Jun. "Tiyu, Shengong, Pianzi" (Physical exercise, supernatural qigong, and swindler). *Renmin Ribao* (People's daily), July 10, 1990.

Liu, Lydia. *Translingual Practice: Literature, National Culture, and Translated Modernity—China, 1900–1937.* Stanford, Calif.: Stanford University Press, 1995.

Liu, Peng. "Yiwei Qigong Aihaozhe De Qingsu" (The pouring out of one qigong fan). *Zhongguo Tiyubao* (Chinese exercise news), February 3, 1990.

Liu, Shikuan. " 'Yuhuangdadi de Nuer'—Zhang Xiangyu Qiren Qishi" ("The daughter of god"—The person and behavior of Zhang Xiangyu). *Falu Yu Shenghuo* (Law and life) 10 (1990): 8–10.

Liu, Tianjun. *Qigong Rujing Zhimen* (The gate to relaxation in qigong practice). Beijing: Renmin Tiyu Chubanshe (People's physical training press), 1990.

——. "Qigong Shinian Fazhan Yipie" (The ten-year development of qigong). *Zhongguo Yiyaobao* (Chinese medicine news), March 28, 1991.

Liu, Xiehe. "Psychiatry in Traditional Chinese Medicine." *British Journal of Psychiatry* 138 (1981): 429–33.

Liu, Xin, *In One's Shadow: An Ethnographic Account of the Condition of Post-reform Rural China.* Berkeley: University of California Press, 2000.

Liu, Xinwu. "Bus Aria." In *Black Walls and Other Stories*, trans. D. Cohn, 15–60. Hong Kong: Rendition, 1990.

Liu, Y. L., W. C. Hsiao, and K. Eggleston. "Equity in Health and Health Care: The Chinese Experience." *Social Science and Medicine* 49, no. 10 (November 1999): 1349–56.

Liu, Y. L., W. C. L. Hsiao, Q. Li, X. Z. Liu, et al. "Transformation Of China's Rural Health Care Financing." *Social Science and Medicine* 41, no. 8 (October 1995): 1085–93.

Liu, Yanchi. *The Essential Book of Traditional Chinese Medicine.* Vol. 1, *Theory.* New York: Columbia University Press, 1988.

Liu, Yuanli, William C. Hsiao, and Karen Eggleston. "Equity in Health and Health Care: The Chinese Experience." *Social Science and Medicine* 49 (1999): 1349–56.

Livingston, Martha and Paul Lowinger. *The Minds of the Chinese People: Mental Health in New China.* Englewood Cliffs, N.J.: Prentice-Hall, 1983.

Lock, Margaret. *East Asian Medicine in Urban Japan: Varieties of Medical Experience.* Berkeley: University of California Press, 1980.

——. "Cultivating the Body: Anthropology and Epistemologies of Bodily Practice and Knowledge." *Annual Review of Anthropology* 22 (1993): 133–55.

——. *Encounters with Aging: Mythologies of Menopause in Japan and North America.* Berkeley: University of California Press, 1993.

Lock, Margaret and Deborah Gordon. *Biomedicine Examined.* Dordrecht: Kluwer Academic, 1988.

Long, Wenyu and Wang Pengling, eds. *Gujin Gongfa Jicui* (Collection of ancient and modern qigong practice methods). Changchun, Jilin Province: Jilin Kexue Jishu Chubanshe (Jilin science and technology press), 1989.

Low, Setha. "Culturally Interpreted Symptoms or Culture-bound Syndromes." *Social Science and Medicine* 21 (1985): 187–97.

——. "The Anthropology of Cities: Imagining and Theorizing the City." *Annual Review of Anthropology* 25 (1996): 383–409.

Lowe, Donald. *The Body in Late Capitalist USA.* Durham, N.C.: Duke University Press, 1996.

Lowe, Lisa. *Immigrant Acts: On Asian American Cultural Politics.* Durham, N.C.: Duke University Press, 1996.

Lu, Shan. "Jianbie Waiqi Da Leiji" (Taking up the challenge of questioning the existence of outside qi). *Falu Yu Shenghuo* (Law and life) 10 (1991): 18–21.

Lu, Xiaobo. *Cadres and Corruption: The Organizational Involution of the Chinese Communist Party.* Stanford, Calif.: Stanford University Press, 2000.

Lu, Xiaobo and Elizabeth J. Perry, eds. *Danwei: The Changing Chinese Workplace in Historical and Comparative Perspective.* Armonk, N.Y.: Sharpe, 1997.

Lu, Xun. *Diary of a Madman and Other Stories.* Trans. William A. Lyell. Honolulu: University of Hawaii Press, 1990.

Ludmerer, Kenneth M. *Time to Heal: American Medical Education from the Turn of the Century to the Era of Managed Care.* Oxford: Oxford University Press, 1999.

Luhrmann, T. M. *Of Two Minds: The Growing Disorder in American Psychiatry.* New York: Knopf, 2000.

Lutz, Tom. *American Nervousness, 1903: An Anecdotal History.* Ithaca: Cornell University Press, 1991.

Lyon, Margot. "Emotion as Mediator of Somatic and Social Process: The Example of Respiration." *Social Perspectives on Emotion* 2 (1994): 83–108.

Lyon, Margot and J. M. Barbalet. "Society's Body: Emotion and the 'Somatization' of Social Theory." In *Embodiment and Experience: The Existential Ground of Culture and Self,* ed. Thomas J. Csordas, 48–66. Cambridge: Cambridge University Press, 1994.

Lynch, Owen. *Divine Passions.* Berkeley: University of California Press, 1990.

McCagg, William O. and Lewis Siegelbaum. *The Disabled in the Soviet Union: Past and Present, Theory and Practice.* Pittsburgh: University of Pittsburgh Press, 1989.

McDonald, Joe. "China Tightens Security on Falun Gong Anniversary." Associated Press, May 13, 2002.

MacDonald, M. *Mystical Bedlam.* Cambridge: Cambridge University Press, 1981.

Mackay, Charles, *Extraordinary Popular Delusions and the Madness of Crowds.* Foreword Andrew Tobias. 1853. Reprint, New York: Harmony, 1980.

McNeill, John T. *A History of the Cure of Souls.* New York: Harper and Row, 1951.

Madsen, Richard. *Morality and Power in a Chinese Village.* Berkeley: University of California Press, 1984.

Malinowski, Bronislaw. *Magic, Science, and Religion and Other Essays.* Glenco, Ill.: Free, 1948.

Mao, Zedong. *Selected Works of Mao Zedong.* Vol. 1. Beijing: Foreign Languages Press, 1965.

Marcus, George E. and Michael M. J. Fischer. *Anthropology as Cultural Critique: An Experimental Moment in the Human Sciences.* Chicago: University of Chicago Press, 1986.

Marsella, Anthony, George DeVos, and Francis Hsu, eds. *Culture and Self.* London: Tavistock, 1985.

Marsella, Anthony and Geoffrey M. White, eds. *Cultural Conceptions of Mental Health and Therapy.* Dordrecht: Reidel, 1982.

Martin, Emily. *The Woman in the Body: A Cultural Analysis of Reproduction.* Boston: Beacon, 1987.

——. "The End of the Body?" *American Ethnologist* 19, no. 1 (February 1992): 121–40.

——. *Flexible Bodies: Tracking Immunity in American Culture from the Days of Polio to the Age of AIDS.* Boston: Beacon, 1994.

Massey, Doreen. "Power Geometry and a Progressive Sense of Place." In *Mapping the Future: Local Culture, Global Change,* ed. J. Bird, B. Curtis, T. Putnam, G. Robertson, and L. Tickner, 59–69. New York: Routledge, 1993.

——. *Space, Place, and Gender.* Minneapolis: University of Minnesota Press, 1994.

Mayer, Jean François. "Sects and New Religious Movements: Questions and Challenges for Armed Forces and National Security." Paper presented at Minorities and Armed Forces II: Ethnic and Religious Minorities Within the Military, Vienna, May 12–15, 1999.

Merleau-Ponty, M. *The Phenomenology of Perception*. Trans. Colin Smith. London: Routledge, 1981.

Meyer, Jeffrey. *The Dragons of Tiananmen: Beijing as Sacred City*. Columbia: University of South Carolina Press, 1991.

Micale, Mark S. and Roy Porter, eds. *Discovering the History of Psychiatry*. New York: Oxford University Press, 1994.

Micollier, Evelyne. "Qigong Groups and Civil Society in P.R. China." *International Institute for Asian Studies Newsletter*, no. 22 (June 2000): 32.

Miller, H. Lyman. *Science and Dissent in Post-Mao China: The Politics of Knowledge*. Seattle: University of Washington Press, 1996.

Miura, Kunio. "The Revival of Qi." In *Taoist Meditation and Longevity Techniques*, ed. Livia Kohn, 331–62. Ann Arbor: Center for Chinese Studies, University of Michigan, 1989.

Moore, R. Laurence (Robert Laurence), *Religious Outsiders and the Making of Americans*. New York: Oxford University Press, 1986.

———. *Selling God: American Religion in the Marketplace of Culture*. New York: Oxford University Press, 1994.

Montgomery, Scott, "Illness and Image in Holistic Discourse: How Alternative Is 'Alternative'?" *Cultural Critique*, no. 25 (fall 1993): 65–89.

Morris, Glenn. *Martial Arts Madness: Light and Dark in the Esoteric Arts*. Berkeley, Calif.: Frog, 1998.

Morris, Rosalind C. *In the Place of Origins: Modernity and Its Mediums in Northern Thailand*. Durham, N.C.: Duke University Press, 2000.

Moyers, Bill D. *Healing and the Mind*. New York: Doubleday, 1993.

Mueggler, Erik. *The Age of Wild Ghosts: Memory, Violence, and Place in Southwest China*. Berkeley: University of California Press, 2001.

Mumford, Lewis. *The Culture of Cities*. New York: Harcourt, Brace 1938.

Munro, Robin. "Synchretic Sects and Secret Societies: Revival in the 1980s." *Chinese Sociology and Anthropology* 21, no. 4 (1989): 3–103.

———. "Judicial Psychiatry in China and Its Political Abuses." *Columbia Journal of Asian Law* 14, no. 1 (spring 2000): 106–20.

———. "Political Psychiatry in Post-Mao China and Its Origins in the Cultural Revolution." *Journal of the American Academy of Psychiatry and the Law* 30, no. 1 (2002): 97–106.

———. "On the Psychiatric Abuse of Falun Gong and Other Dissenters in China: A Reply to Stone, Hickling, Kleinman, and Lee." *Journal of the American Academy of Psychiatry and the Law* 30, no. 2 (2002): 266–74.

Nader, Laura. "Up the Anthropologist: Perspectives Gained from Studying Up." In *Reinventing Anthropology*, ed. D. Hymes, 285–311. New York: Pantheon, 1972.

———, ed. *Naked Science: Anthropological Inquiry into Boundaries, Power, and Knowledge*. New York: Routledge, 1996.

Nakayama, Shigeru and Nathan Sivin, eds. *Chinese Science: Explorations of an Ancient Tradition*. Cambridge, Mass.: MIT Press, 1973.

Naquin, Susan. *Millenarian Rebellion in China: The Eight Trigrams Uprising of 1813.* New Haven: Yale University Press, 1976.

———. *Shantung Rebellion: The Wang Lun Uprising of 1774.* New Haven: Yale University Press, 1981.

———. *Peking: Temples and City Life, 1400–1900.* Berkeley: University of California Press, 2000.

Naquin, Susan and Chun-fang Yu. *Pilgrims and Sacred Sites in China.* Berkeley: University of California Press, 1992.

Narayan, Kirin. "How Native Is a 'Native' Anthropologist?" In *Situated Lives: Gender and Culture in Everyday Life.* Ed. Louise Lamphere, Helene Ragone, and Patricia Zavella, 23–41. New York: Routledge, 1997.

"Nation's Mentally Ill Need More Care." *China Daily*, November 27, 2000.

Navaro-Yashin, Yael. *Faces of the State: Secularism and Public Life in Turkey.* Princeton: Princeton University Press, 2002.

Needham, Joseph. *Science and Civilisation in China.* 7 vols. Cambridge: Cambridge University Press, 1954–2000.

———. *Science in Traditional China: A Comparative Perspective.* Cambridge: Harvard University Press, 1981.

Ng, Beng-Yeong. "Qigong-induced Mental Disorders: A Review." *Australian and New Zealand Journal Of Psychiatry* 33, no. 2 (April 1999): 197–206.

Ng, Vivien W. *Madness in Late Imperial China: From Illness to Deviance.* Norman: University of Oklahoma Press, 1990.

Ning, Yuan, ed. *Zhongguo Dangdai Qigong Jinglun* (Discussion of contemporary Chinese qigong). Beijing: Renmin Tiyu Chubanshe (People's physical training press), 1990.

Nomora, Naoki. *Ethnography of a Japanese Mental Hospital.* Ph.D. diss., Stanford University, 1987.

O'Neill, John. *Five Bodies: The Human Shape of Modern Society.* Ithaca: Cornell University Press, 1985.

Ong, Aihwa. *Spirits of Resistance and Capitalist Discipline: Factory Women in Malaysia.* Albany: SUNY Press, 1987.

———. *Flexible Citizenship: The Cultural Logics of Transnationality.* Durham, N.C.: Duke University Press, 1999.

Ong, Aihwa and Don Nonini, eds. *Ungrounded Empires: The Cultural Politics of Modern Chinese Transnationalism.* New York: Routledge, 1997.

Ong, Han. *Fixer Chao.* New York: Farrar, Straus and Giroux, 2001.

Orleans, Leo A. *Science in Contemporary China.* Stanford, Calif.: Stanford University Press, 1980.

Ots, Thomas. *Medizin und Heilung in China: Annaherungen an die Traditionelle Chinesische Medizin.* Berlin: Dietrich Reimer, 1987.

———. "The Silent Body, The Loud Leib: Mind Versus Life in Chinese Cathartic Healing." In *Embodiment and Experience: The Existential Ground of Culture and Self,* ed. Thomas Csordas, 116–36. Cambridge: Cambridge University Press, 1994.

Overmyer, Daniel L. *Folk Buddhist Religion: Dissenting Sects in Late Traditional China*. Cambridge: Harvard University Press, 1976.

——. *Religions of China: The World as a Living System*. San Francisco: Harper and Row, 1986.

——. *Precious Volumes: An Introduction to Chinese Sectarian Scriptures from the Sixteenth and Seventeenth Centuries*. Cambridge: Harvard University Asia Center, 1999; distributed by Harvard University Press.

Ownby, David. *Brotherhoods and Secret Societies in Early and Mid-Qing China: The Formation of a Tradition*. Stanford, Calif.: Stanford University Press, 1996.

——. "Imperial Fantasies: The Chinese Communists and Peasant Rebellions." *Comparative Studies in Society and History* 43, no. 1 (January 2001): 65–91.

Ownby, David and Mary Somers Heidhues, eds. *"Secret Societies" Reconsidered: Perspectives on the Social History of Modern South China and Southeast Asia*. Armonk, N.Y.: Sharpe, 1993.

Palmer, David. "Qigong, Scientism, and Millenialism." Paper presented at "Chinese Millenialism in Comparative Perspective," Harvard University/Boston University, April 28–29, 2002.

Pan, Philip. "Five People Set Themselves Afire in China." *Washington Post*, January 24, 2001, A16.

Pas, Julian, ed. *The Turning of the Tide: Religion in China Today*. Hong Kong: Oxford University Press, 1989.

Pearson, Veronica. *Mental Health Care in China: State Policies, Professional Services and Family Responsibilities*. London: Gaskell, 1995.

Pearson, V. and M. R. Phillips. "The Social Context of Psychiatric Rehabilitation in China." *British Journal of Psychiatry* 165, supp. 24 (August 1994): 11–18.

Penny, Benjamin. "Qigong, Daoism, and Science: Some Contexts for the Qigong Boom." In *Modernization of the Chinese Past*, ed. Mabel Lee and A. D. Syrokomla-Stefanowska, 166–79. Canberra, Australia: Wild Peony, 1993.

Perry, Elizabeth J. *Shanghai on Strike: The Politics of Chinese Labor*. Stanford, Calif.: Stanford University Press, 1993.

——. "Challenging the Mandate of Heaven—Popular Protest in Modern China." *Critical Asian Studies* 33, no. 2 (June 2001): 163–80.

Perry, Elizabeth J. and Ellen V. Fuller. "China's Long March to Democracy." *World Policy Journal* 7, no. 3 (fall 1991): 663–85.

Perry, Elizabeth J. and Christine Wong, eds. *The Political Economy of Reform in Post-Mao China*. Cambridge: Harvard University Press, 1985.

Peterson, Dale, ed. *A Mad People's History of Madness*. Pittsburgh: University of Pittsburgh Press, 1982.

Petzold, Matthias, ed. "Psychology in Contemporary China, Part I." *Chinese Sociology and Anthropology* 12, no. 3 (spring 1980): 3–126.

Phillips, M. R. "The Transformation of China's Mental Health Service." *China Journal* 39 (January 1998): 1–36.

Phillips, M. R., Y. Y. Li, T. S. Stroup, and L. H. Xin. "Causes of Schizophrenia Reported by Patients' Family Members in China." *British Journal of Psychiatry* 177 (July 2000): 20–25.

Phillips, M. R., H. Q. Liu, and Y. P. Zhang. "Suicide and Social Change in China." *Culture, Medicine, and Psychiatry* 23, no. 1 (1999): 25–50.

Phillips, M. R., S. H. Lu, and R. W. Wang. "Economic Reforms and the Acute Inpatient Care of Patients with Schizophrenia: The Chinese Experience." *American Journal of Psychiatry* 154, no. 9 (September 1997): 1228–34.

Phillips, Michael R., Veronica Pearson, and Ruiwen Wang, eds. "Psychiatric Rehabilitation in China: Models for Change in a Changing Society." *British Journal of Psychiatry* 165, supp. 24 (August 1994).

Picone, Mary. "The Ghost in the Machine: Religious Healing and Representations of the Body in Japan." In *Fragments for a History of the Human Body*, ed. Michel Feher, Ramona Naddaff, and Nadia Tazi, 466–89. Cambridge, Mass.: MIT Press, 1988.

Pieke, Frank. *The Ordinary and the Extraordinary: An Anthropological Study of Chinese Reform and the 1989 People's Movement in Beijing.* London: Kegan Paul International, 1996.

Pile, Steve and Michael Keith, eds. *Geographies of Resistance.* London: Routledge, 1997.

Pomfret, John. "China Holds 40 Foreign Falun Gong Protesters: Use of Westerners Marks New Tactic." *Washington Post*, February 15, 2002, A26.

Porkert, Manfred. *The Theoretical Foundations of Chinese Medicine: Systems of Correspondence.* Cambridge, Mass.: MIT Press, 1974.

Porter, Dorothy and Roy Porter. *Doctors, Politics and Society: Historical Essays.* Amsterdam: Rodopi, 1993.

Porter, Roy. *A Social History of Madness: The World through the Eyes of the Insane.* London: Weidenfeld and Nicolson, 1987.

Pye, Lucien. *The Spirit of Chinese Politics: A Psychocultural Study of the Authority Crisis in Political Development.* Cambridge, Mass.: MIT Press, 1968.

Quesada, James. *Contested Lives, Contested Territories: An Ethnography of Polarization, Distress, and Suffering in Post-Sandinista Nicaragua.* Ph.D. diss., University of California Berkeley—San Francisco, 1994.

Reed, Louis S. *The Healing Cult: A Study of Sectarian Medical Practice—Its Extent, Causes, and Control.* Chicago, University of Chicago Press, 1932.

Rhodes, Lorna A. *Emptying Beds: The Work of an Emergency Psychiatric Unit.* Berkeley: University of California Press, 1991.

Rival, Laura, ed. *The Social Life of Trees: Anthropological Perspectives on Tree Symbolism.* Oxford: Berg, 1998.

Robbins, Thomas, William C. Shepherd, and James McBride, eds. *Cults, Culture, and the Law: Perspectives on New Religious Movements.* Chico, Calif.: Scholars, 1985.

Robinet, Isabelle. *Taoism: Growth of a Religion.* Stanford, Caluf.: Stanford University Press, 1997.

Rofel, Lisa. *Other Modernities: Gendered Yearnings in China After Socialism.* Berkeley: University of California Press, 1999.

Rose, Gillian. *Feminism and Geography: The Limits of Geographical Knowledge*. Cambridge: Polity, 1993.

Rose, Nikolas S. *Governing the Soul: The Shaping of the Private Self*. London: Routledge, 1990.

——. *Inventing Our Selves: Psychology, Power, and Personhood*. Cambridge: Cambridge University Press, 1996.

Rose, Nikolas S. and Peter Miller, eds. *The Power of Psychiatry*. Cambridge: Polity; New York: Blackwell, 1986.

Rosenzweig, Roy and Elizabeth Blackmar. *The Park and the People: A History of Central Park*. Ithaca: Cornell University Press, 1992.

Roth, Harold David. *Original Tao: Inward Training (nei-yeh) and the Foundations of Taoist Mysticism*. New York: Columbia University Press, 1999.

Saich, Tony. *China's Science Policy in the 80s*. Manchester: Manchester University Press, 1989.

Sapir, Edward. *Selected Writings of Edward Sapir in Language, Culture, and Personality*. Ed. David G. Mandelbaum. Berkeley: University of California Press, 1985.

Sassen, Saskia. *Cities in a World Economy*. Thousand Oaks, Calif.: Pine Forge, 1994.

——. *Globalization and Its Discontents: Essays on the New Mobility of People and Money*. New York: New, 1998.

Schauble, John. "China Puts Square Suicides on TV." *The Age*, February 1, 2001.

Schechter, Danny. *Falun Gong's Challenge to China: Spiritual Practice or "Evil Cult"?* New York: Akashic, 2000.

Schein, Louisa. *Minority Rules: The Miao and the Feminine in China's Cultural Politics*. Durham, N.C.: Duke University Press, 2000.

Scheper-Hughes, Nancy. *Saints, Scholars, and Schizophrenics: Mental Illness in Rural Ireland*. Berkeley: University of California Press, 1979.

——. *Death Without Weeping: The Violence of Everyday Life in Brazil*. Berkeley: University of California Press, 1992.

Scheper-Hughes, Nancy and Margaret Lock. "Speaking Truth to Illness: Metaphors, Reification, and a Pedagogy for Patients." *Medical Anthropology Quarterly* 17, no. 5 (1986): 137–40.

——. "The Mindful Body: A Prolegomenon to Future Work in Medical Anthropology." *Medical Anthropology Quarterly* 1 (1987): 6–41.

Scheper-Hughes, Nancy and Anne M. Lovell, eds. *Psychiatry Inside Out: Selected Writings of Franco Basaglia*. New York: Columbia University Press, 1987.

Schipper, Kristofer. *The Taoist Body*. Trans. Karen C. Duval. Berkeley, Calif.: University of California Press, 1993.

Scott, James. *Domination and the Arts of Resistance: Hidden Transcripts*. New Haven: Yale University Press, 1990.

——. *Seeing Like a State: How Certain Schemes to Improve the Human Condition Have Failed*. New Haven: Yale University Press, 1998.

Scull, Andrew. *The Social Organization of Insanity in Nineteenth-Century England*. London: Allen Lane, 1979.

Sedgwick, Peter. *Psycho Politics: Laing, Foucault, Goffman, Szasz, and the Future of Mass Psychiatry.* New York: Harper and Row, 1982.

Sennett, Richard. *The Uses of Disorder: Personal Identity and City Life.* New York: Norton, 1992.

———. *Flesh and Stone: The Body and the City in Western Civilization.* New York: Norton, 1994.

Shaara, Lila and Andrew Strathern. "A Preliminary Analysis of the Relationship Between Altered States of Consciousness, Healing, and Social Structure." *American Anthropologist* 94, no. 1 (March 1992): 145–60.

Shahar, Meir. *Crazy Ji: Chinese Religion and Popular Literature.* Cambridge: Harvard University Asia Center and Harvard University Press, 1998.

Shahar, Meir and Rob Weller, eds. *Unruly Gods: Divinity and Society in China.* Honolulu: University of Hawaii Press.

Shan, Huaihai. "Qigong Piancha Yukuan Wenhua Jingshen Yixue" (Qigong deviation and cross-cultural mental health study). *Jiankang Ribao* (Health daily), May 16, 1990.

Shan, Huaihai, Yan Wenwei, and Yan Heqin. "Dai Gong Bao Gao Zhong De Jing Shen Yi Xue Wen Ti" (The mental health issue in the lectures with qigong). *Jiankang Ribao* (Health daily), August 4, 1990.

Sharp, Lesley. "Possessed and Dispossessed Youth: Spirit Possession of School Children in Northwest Madagascar." *Culture, Medicine, and Psychiatry* 14, no. 3 (1991): 339–64.

———. *The Possessed and the Dispossessed: Spirits, Identity, and Power in a Madagascar Migrant Town.* Berkeley, Calif.: University of California Press, 1993.

Shen, Yucun. *Jing Shen Bing Xue* (Psychiatry). Beijing: Ren Min Wei Sheng Chu Ban She (People's health press), 1980.

Shorter, Edward. *From Paralysis to Fatigue: A History of Psychosomatic Illness in the Modern Era.* New York: Free; Toronto: Maxwell Macmillan, 1992.

———. *From the Mind into the Body: The Cultural Origins of Psychosomatic Symptoms.* New York: Maxwell Macmillan International, 1994.

———. *A History of Psychiatry: From the Era of the Asylum to the Age of Prozac.* New York: Wiley, 1997.

Showalter, Elaine. *Hystories: Hysterical Epidemics and Modern Culture.* New York: Columbia University Press, 1997.

Shue, Vivienne. *The Reach of the State: Sketches of the Chinese Body Politic.* Stanford, Calif.: Stanford University Press, 1988.

———. "State Legitimization in China: The Challenge of Popular Religion." Paper presented at the annual meeting of the American Political Science Association, Boston, 2001.

Sidel, Victor W. and Ruth Sidel. *Serve the People: Observations on Medicine in the People's Republic of China.* New York: Josiah Macy Jr. Foundation, 1973.

Simmel, Georg. "The Metropolis and Mental Life." In *The Sociology of Georg Simmel,* ed. and trans. Kurt H. Wolff, 409–24. New York: Free, 1964.

Sigurdson, Jon. *Technology and Science in the People's Republic of China: An Introduction.* Oxford: Pergamon, 1980.

Simon, Denis Fred and Goldman, Merle, eds. *Science and Technology in Post-Mao China.* Cambridge: Harvard University Press, 1989.

Singer, Margaret, with Janja Lalich. *Cults in Our Midst.* San Francisco: Jossey-Bass, 1995.

Siu, Helen. "Socialist Peddlers and Princes in a Chinese Market Town." *American Ethnologist* 16, no.2 (May 1989): 195–212.

Sivin, Nathan. *Medicine, Philosophy and Religion in Ancient China: Researches and Reflections.* Aldershot: Variorum, 1995a.

——. *Science in Ancient China: Researches and Reflections.* Aldershot: Variorum, 1995b.

Skinner, G. William. "Marketing and Social Structure in Rural China." *Journal of Asian Studies* 24 (1964–65): 3–43, 195–228, 363–399.

——. "Cities and the Hierarchy of Local Systems." In *The City in Late Imperial China*, ed. G. William Skinner, 275–351. Stanford, Calif.: Stanford University Press, 1977.

Smith, Christopher J. "Modernization and Health Care in Contemporary China." *Health and Place* 4, no. 2 (1998): 125–39.

Soja, Edward. *Postmodern Geographies.* New York: Routledge, 1989.

Solinger, Dorothy. *Contesting Citizenship in Urban China: Peasant Migrants, the State, and the Logic of the Market.* Berkeley: University of California Press, 1999.

Sorell, Tom. *Scientism: Philosophy and the Infatuation with Science.* London: Routledge, 1991.

Spence, Jonathan D. *The Memory Palace of Matteo Ricci.* New York: Viking Penguin, 1984.

——. *The Question of Hu.* New York: Vintage, 1988.

——. *The Search for Modern China.* New York: Norton, 1990.

——. *God's Chinese Son: The Taiping Heavenly Kingdom of Hong Xiuquan.* New York: Norton, 1996.

Spiegel, David. *Dissociation: Culture, Mind, and Body.* Washington, D.C.: American Psychiatric, 1994.

Stewart, K. and S. Harding. "Bad Endings: American Apocalypsis." *Annual Review of Anthropology* 28 (1999): 285–310.

Stoller, Paul. *Fusion of the Worlds: An Ethnography of Possession Among the Songhay of Niger.* Chicago: University of Chicago Press, 1989.

——. *Embodying Colonial Memories: Spirit Possession, Power, and the Hauka in West Africa.* New York: Routledge, 1995.

——. *Sensuous Scholarship.* Philadelphia: University of Pennsylvania Press, 1997.

Strand, David. *Rickshaw Beijing: City People and Politics in the 1920s.* Berkeley: University of California Press, 1989.

Strickmann, Michel. *Chinese Magical Medicine.* Ed. Bernard Faure. Stanford, Calif.: Stanford University Press, 2002.

Sun, Longji. "Contemporary Chinese Culture: Structure and Emotionality." *Australian Journal of Chinese Affairs* 26 (1991): 1–41.

Szasz, Thomas. *The Manufacture of Madness*. London: Routledge&, 1971.

Tai, Hue-Tam Ho. *Millenarianism and Peasant Politics in Vietnam*. Cambridge: Harvard University Press, 1983.

Tambiah, Stanley Jeyaraja. *Magic, Science, Religion, and the Scope of Rationality*. Cambridge: Cambridge University Press, 1990.

——. *Leveling Crowds: Ethnonationalist Conflicts and Collective Violence in South Asia*. Berkeley: University of California Press, 1996.

Tang, Xiaobing. *Global Space and the Nationalist Discourse of Modernity: The Historical Thinking of Liang Qichao*. Stanford, Calif.: Stanford University Press, 1996.

Taussig, Michael. *Shamanism, Colonialism, and the Wild Man*. Chicago: University of Chicago Press, 1987.

——. *The Nervous System*. New York: Routledge, 1992.

Thurston, Anne F. *Enemies of the People*. New York: Knopf, 1987.

Tseng, W. S. and David Wu, eds. *Chinese Culture and Mental Health*. Orlando: Academic, 1986.

Tseng, Wen Shing, Hu Di, Keisuke Ebata, Jin Hsu, and Cui Yuhua. "Diagnostic Pattern for Neuroses in China, Japan, and the United States." *American Journal of Psychiatry* 143, no. 3 (1986): 1010–14.

Tseng, Wen-Shing and John McDermott. *Culture, Mind, and Therapy*. New York: Brunner-Mazel, 1981.

Tsing, Anna L. *In the Realm of the Diamond Queen*. Princeton: Princeton University Press, 1993.

Tu, Wei-ming, ed. "China in Transformation." *Daedalus* 122, no. 2(spring 1993): 7–24.

——. *The Living Tree: The Changing Meaning of Being Chinese Today*. Stanford, Calif.: Stanford University Press, 1994.

Tuan, Yi-fu. *Space and Place: The Perspective of Experience*. Minneapolis: University of Minnesota Press, 1977.

——. *Landscapes of Fear*. Minneapolis: University of Minnesota Press, 1979.

——. *Segmented Worlds and Self: Group Life and Individual Consciousness*. Minneapolis: University of Minnesota Press, 1982.

——. *The Good Life*. Madison: University of Wisconsin Press, 1986.

Turner, Bryan S. *Medical Power and Social Knowledge*. London: Sage, 1987.

——. *Orientalism, Postmodernism, and Globalism*. London: Routledge, 1994.

——. *The Body and Society: Explorations in Social Theory*. 2d ed. London: Sage, 1996.

Turner, Bryan S. and Colin Samson. *Medical Power and Social Knowledge*. 2d ed. London: Sage, 1995.

Turner, Victor and E. M. Bruner, eds. *The Anthropology of Experience*. Urbana: University of Illinois Press, 1986.

Unschuld, Paul. *Medical Ethics in Imperial China: A Study in Historical Anthropology*. Berkeley: University of California Press, 1979.

——. *Medicine in China: A History of Ideas.* Berkeley: University of California Press, 1985.

——. *Medicine in China: A History of Pharmaceutics.* Berkeley: University of California Press, 1986.

——, ed. *Medicine in China: The Nan-ching—Classic of Difficult Issues.* Berkeley: University of California Press, 1986.

Urry, John. *Consuming Places.* London: Routledge, 1995.

Verdery, Katherine. *What Was Socialism, and What Comes Next?* Princeton: Princeton University Press, 1996.

Vieth, Ilza. *Huangti Neijing Suwen: The Yellow Emperor's Canon of Medicine.* San Francisco: University of California Press, 1978.

Wakeman, Frederic E., Jr. *History and Will: Philosophical Perspectives of Mao Tse-tung's Thought.* Berkeley: University of California Press, 1973.

——. *The Fall of Imperial China.* New York: Free, 1975.

——. *The Great Enterprise: The Manchu Reconstruction of Imperial Order in Seventeenth-Century China.* Berkeley: University of California Press, 1985.

——. *Policing Shanghai, 1927–1937.* Berkeley: University of California Press, 1995.

——. *Strangers at the Gate: Social Disorder in South China, 1839–1861.* Berkeley: University of California Press, 1997.

Waley-Cohen, Joanna. *The Sextants of Beijing: Global Currents in Chinese History.* New York: Norton, 1999.

Wallace, Anthony F. C. *Culture and Personality.* New York: Random House, 1961.

Wang, Bingcai and Niu Kezhen, eds. *Shequ Jingshen Yixue Zhishi Wenda* (Questions and answers on community mental health knowledge). Zhaoyuan, Shandong Province: Zhaoyuan Jingshen Bingyuan (Zhaoyuan County Mental Health Hospital), 1989.

Wang, Erfeng and Xiao Zhou. *Jin Dan* (Chemical pellet). Beijing: Zhongguo Funu Chubanshe (Chinese women press), 1989.

Wang, Hui. "The Fate of 'Mr. Science' in China: The Concept of Science and Its Application in Modern Chinese Thought." *Positions* 3, no. 1 (spring 1995): 1–68.

Wang, Jing. *High Culture Fever: Politics, Aesthetics and Ideology in Deng's China.* Berkeley: University of California Press, 1996.

Wang, K. Chi-min and Lien-Teh Wu. *History of Chinese Medicine; Being a Chronicle of Medical Happenings in China from Ancient Times to the Present Period.* 2d ed. Shanghai: National Quarantine Service, 1936. Reprint, New York: AMS, 1973.

Wang, Songling. *Zhongguo Qigong De Shi, Li, Fa* (The history, theory and method of Chinese qigong). Beijing: Huaxia Chubanshe, 1989.

Wang, Yeu-Farn. *China's Science and Technology Policy, 1949–1989.* Aldershot: Avebury, 1993.

Wang, Zhengfan. "Qigong Lian Budang, Jingshen Yaocuo Luan" (Inappropriate practicing of qigong can cause mental illness). *Jiankang Ribao* (Health daily), January 31, 1989.

Wasserstrom, Jeffrey N. *Student Protests in Twentieth-Century China: The View from Shanghai.* Stanford, Calif.: Stanford University Press, 1991.

Wasserstrom, Jeffrey N. and Elizabeth J. Perry. *Popular Protestant Political Culture in Modern China: Learning from 1989.* Boulder, Colo.: Westview, 1992.

Watson, Sophie and Katherine Gibson. *Postmodern Cities and Spaces.* Oxford: Basil Blackwell, 1995.

Weber, Max. *The Protestant Ethic and the Spirit of Capitalism.* Trans. Talcott Parsons. 1992. Reprint, London: Routledge, 1994.

Weber, Max. *The Religion of China.* Trans. Talcott Parsons. New York: Macmillan, 1951.

Weller, Robert P. *Resistance, Chaos, and Control in China: Taiping Rebels, Taiwanese Ghosts, and Tiananmen.* Seattle: University of Washington Press, 1994.

——. "Living at the Edge: Religion, Capitalism, and the End of the Nation-State in Taiwan." *Public Culture* 12, no. 2 (2000): 477–98.

Wen, Jung-Kwang. "The Hall of Dragon Metamorphoses—A Unique, Indigenous Asylum for Chronic Mental Patients In Taiwan." *Culture, Medicine, and Psychiatry* 14, no. 1 (1990): 1–19.

Wen-hsin, Yeh, ed. *Becoming Chinese: Passages to Modernity and Beyond.* Berkeley: University of California Press, 2000.

White, Sydney. "Deciphering 'Integrated Chinese and Western Medicine' in the Rural Lijiang Basin: State Policy and Local Practice(s) in Socialist China." *Social Science and Medicine* 49, no. 10 (November 1999): 1333–47.

Whyte, Martin K. *Small Groups and Political Rituals in China.* Berkeley: University of California Press, 1974.

Whyte, Martin K. and William L. Parish. *Urban Life in Contemporary China.* Chicago: University of Chicago Press, 1984.

Williams, Raymond. *The Country and the City.* New York: Oxford University Press, 1973.

——. *Resources of Hope: Culture, Democracy, Socialism.* London: Verso, 1989.

Wilson, Elizabeth. *The Sphinx in the City: Urban Life, the Control of Disorder, and Women.* Berkeley: University of California Press, 1991.

Winter, Alison. *Mesmerized: Powers of Mind in Victorian Britain.* Chicago: University of Chicago Press, 1998.

Wolf, Arthur P. and Emily Ahern, eds. *Religion and Ritual in Chinese Society.* Stanford, Calif.: Stanford University Press, 1974.

Wong, V. C. and S. W. Chiu. "Health-Care Reforms in the People's Republic of China—Strategies and Social Implications." *Journal of Management in Medicine* 12, no. 4 (1998): 270–86.

Wong, John and William T. Liu. *The Mystery of China's Falun Gong: Its Rise and Its Sociological Implications.* Singapore: World Scientific Publishing, 1999.

Wortis, Joseph, *Soviet Psychiatry.* Baltimore, Williams and Wilkins, 1950.

Wu, Caiyun and Xu Peixi. "Qigong Nengguo Diaodong Qianyishi" (Qigong can motivate the subconsciousness). *Jiankang Ribao* (Health daily), July 7, 1990.

Wu, Y. R. "China's Health Care Sector in Transition: Resources, Demand and Reforms." *Health Policy* 39, no. 2 (February 1997): 137–52.

Xing, Sishao. "Shi Xuanchuan Qigong, Haishi Xuanchuan Mixin" (Do they propagate qigong or spread superstition?). *Jiankang Ribao* (Health daily), December 16, 1990.

Xu, Jian. "Body, Discourse, and the Cultural Politics of Contemporary Chinese Qigong." *Journal of Asian Studies* 58, no. 4 (November 1999): 961–91.

Xu, Qi. "Yan Xin Da Wenlu" (The record of questions and answers about qigong by Yan Xin). *Zhongguo Tiyubao* (Chinese exercise news), December 17, 1989.

Yan, Heqin. "The Necessity of Retaining the Diagnostic Concept of Neurasthenia." *Culture, Medicine, and Psychiatry* 13, no. 2 (1989): 139–45.

Yan, Renxi and Yan Jianjun, eds. *Qigong Yongyu Shouce* (Handbook of qigong phraseology). Beijing: Zhongguo Yiyao Keji Chubanshe (Chinese medical technology press), 1990.

Yan, Yunxiang. *The Flow of Gifts: Reciprocity and Social Networks in a Chinese Village.* Stanford, Calif.: Stanford University Press, 1996.

Yang, Bo. *The Ugly Chinaman and the Crisis of Chinese Culture.* Trans. and ed. Don J. Cohn and Jing Qing. North Sydney: Allen and Unwin, 1992.

Yang, Ching-kun. *The Chinese Family in the Communist Revolution.* Cambridge, Mass.: MIT Press, 1969a.

——. *Religion in Chinese Society: A Study of Contemporary Social Functions of Religion and Some of Their Historical Factors.* Berkeley: University of California Press, 1969b.

Yang, Desen (Young, Derson), ed. *Zhongguo Jingshen Jibing Zhenduan Biaozhun Yu Anli* (Chinese criterion of mental illness diagnosis and case studies). Changsha, Hunan Province: Hunan Daxue Chubanshe (Hunan university press), 1989.

Yang, Jwing-Ming. *Qigong, The Secret of Youth: Da Mo's Muscle/Tendon Changing and Marrow/Brain Washing Classics.* Jamaica Plain, Mass.: Yang's Martial Arts Association, 2000.

Yang, Mayfairs Mei-Hui. *Gifts, Favors, and Banquets: The Art of Social Relationships in China.* Ithaca: Cornell University Press, 1994.

——, ed. *Spaces of Their Own: Women's Public Sphere in Transnational China.* Minneapolis: University of Minnesota Press, 1999.

Yang, Yu. "Zhe Jiuiing Shi Zenme Huishi?" (What is this about?). *Zhongguo Tiyubao* (Chinese exercise news), June 3, 1990.

Yin, Kou, Wen Qu, and Zi Mu, eds. *Lian Qigong Zhe Jie: Zouhuo Rumo* (Warning the qigong practitioner: Qigong deviation). Chengdu, Sichuan Province: Chengdu Keji Daxue Chubanshe (Chengdu technology university press), 1990.

Young, Allan. *The Harmony of Illusions.* Princeton: Princeton University Press, 1997.

Young, Derson and Mingyan Chang. "Psychiatry in the People's Republic of China." *Comprehensive Psychiatry* 24, no. 5 (1983): 431–38.

Yu, Q. Y. *The Implementation of China's Science and Technology Policy.* Westport, Conn.: Quorum, 1999.

Yuasa, Yasuo. *The Body: Toward an Eastern Mind-Body Theory.* Trans. Nagatomo Shigenori and Thomas P. Kasulis. Albany: SUNY Press, 1987.

——. *The Body, Self-Cultivation, and Ki-Energy.* Trans. Shigenori Nagatomo and Monte S. Hull. Albany: SUNY Press, 1993.

Yue, Gang. *The Mouth That Begs: Hunger, Cannibalism, and the Politics of Eating in Modern China.* Durham, N.C.: Duke University Press, 1999.

Zhang, Honglin. "Wei Qigong Zhongzhong" (Many kinds of false qigong). *Falu Yu Shenghuo* (Law and life) 10 (1990): 11–16.

Zhang, Honglin and Hu Weiguo. "Qigong Duanlian You Naxie Tedian" (What are the characteristics of qigong practice). *Zhongguo Tiyubao* (Chinese physical training news), June 17, 1990a.

———. "Weishenme Shuo Qigong Shi Yiliao Baojian Yundong De Fangfa, Kexue He Yishu" (Why say qigong is the method, science, and art of medical care). *Zhongguo Tiyubao* (Chinese exercise news), June 24, 1990b.

———. "Li Daiming Yishi Ruje Kandai Qigong De?" (How ancient and modern famous doctors view qigong?). *Zhongguo Tiyubao* (Chinese exercise news), August 5, 1990c.

———. "Qigong Yu Yiban De Tiyu Duanlian Youhe Yitong" (Similarity and difference between qigong and general physical exercise). *Zhongguo Tiyubao* (Chinese exercise news), September 16, 1990d.

Zhang, Li. *Strangers in the City: Reconfigurations of Space, Power, and Social Networks Within China's Floating Population.* Stanford, Calif.: Stanford University Press, 2001.

Zhang, Mingwu and Sun Xingyuan. *Chinese Qigong Therapy.* Jinan, PRC: Shandong Science and Technology Press, 1988.

Zhang, M. Y., H. Q. Yan, and M. R. Phillips. "Community-Based Psychiatric Rehabilitation in Shanghai: Facilities, Services, Outcome, and Culture-Specific Characteristics." *British Journal of Psychiatry* 165, supp. 24 (August 1994): 70–79.

Zhang, Rongming. *Zhongguo Gudai Qigong Yu Xianqin Zhexue* (Chinese ancient qigong and ancient philosophy). Shanghai: Shanghai Renmin Chubanshe (Shanghai people's press), 1987.

Zhang, Tongling. *Qigong Chupian* (Qigong emergent deviation). Beijing: People's Health Press, 1997.

Zhang, Wenjiang and Chang Jin. *Zhongguo Chuantong Qigongxue Cidian* (The dictionary of traditional Chinese qigong). Daiyuan, Shanxi Province: Shanxi Renmen Chubanshe (Shanxi people's press), 1989.

Zhang, Xin Xin and Sang Ye. *Chinese Lives.* Ed. W. J. F. Jenner and Delia Davin. New York: Pantheon, 1987.

Zhang, Yanghou. *"Da Qigong Shi" Pianshu Jiemi* (Revealing the deceitful trick of the "great qigong master"). Beijing: Falu Chubanshe (Law press), 1991.

Zhang, Yingjin. *The City in Modern Chinese Literature and Film: Configurations of Space, Time, and Gender.* Stanford, Calif.: Stanford University Press, 1996.

Zhang, Zhaozhi. "Wuo Du 'Yan Xin Baogao' " (I read the "report of Yan Xin"). *Qigong Yu Kexue* (Qigong and sciences), no. 9 (1989): 35.

Zhen, Shi. "Daigong Jiangke Mimi Hecai" (What's the secret of lecturing with the body carrying qigong). *Beijing Ribao* (Beijing daily), November 4, 1989.

Zhen, Shiyin. "Youxie Ren Buyilian Qigong" (Some people are not suitable for practicing qigong). *Beijing Wan Bao* (Beijing evening news), April 18, 1990a.

——. "Jinfang Liangong 'Zouhuo Rumo' " (Be careful of "the deviation of qigong"). *Jiankang Ribao* (Health daily), May 17, 1990b.

——. "Zai Xuxu Zhongiian Aode Linghun" (The soul is suffering nihilism). *Jiankang Ribao* (Health daily), June 9, 1990c.

——. "Ermei Qigong Cai Haikou Gongyuan Chuanshou" (The lessons of ermei qigong will be given at Haikou Park). *Hainan Ribao* (Hainan daily), August 11, 1989d.

——. " 'Shenguai Qigong' Bushi Qigong" ("Mystical qigong" is not real qigong). *Cankao Xiaoxi* (Reference news), September 8, 1990e.

——. "Liangong Zouhuo Rumo Zuanjin Ditie Dongnei" (The qigong deviant went to the subway line). *Beijing Wanbao* (Beijing evening news), September 9, 1990f.

——. "Xinxiang Tiyu De Bao Jinliang" (Bao Jinliang's heart is toward the physical training). *Beijing Ribao* (Beijing daily), September 9, 1990g.

Zhi, Fa. "Zhang Xiangyu Shi Zhibing Haishi Hairen" (Is Zhang Xiangyu curing patients or is she doing harm to people?). *Jiankang Ribao* (Health daily), April 19, 1990a.

——. "Yieban Fagong Ji" (Sending the power of qigong at midnight). *Jiankang Ribao* (Health daily), May 26, 1990b.

——. "Shenlan Yu Yuzhouyu" (Supernatural cable and heteroglossia). *Wenhui Bao* (Wenhui news), June 21, 1990c.

——. "Guanyu Zhang Xiangyu Yizi 'Ziran Zhongxin Gong' De Diaocha Zhiyi" (The investigation on Zhang Xiangyu's qigong: Part one). *Jiankang Ribao* (Health daily), July 12, 1990d.

——. "Guanyu Zhang Xiangyu Yiqi 'Ziran Zhongxin Gong' De Diaocha Zhier" (The investigation on Zhang Xiangyu's qigong: Part two). *Jiankang Ribao* (Health daily), July 14, 1990e.

——. "Guanyu Zhang Xiangyu Yiqi 'Ziran Zhongxin Gong' De Diaocha Zhisi" (The investigation on Zhang Xiangyu's qigong: Part four"). *Jiankang Ribao* (Health daily), July 28, 1990f.

——. "Guanyu Zhang Xiangyu Yizi Ziran Zhongxin Gong' De Diaocha Zhiwu" (The investigation on Zhang Xiangyu's qigong: Part five). *Jiankang Ribao* (Health daily), July 29, 1990g.

Zhong, Youbin. *Zhongguo Xinli Fenxi* (Chinese psychoanalysis). Shenyang, Liaoning Province: Liaoning Renmin Chubanshe (Liaoning people's press), 1988.

Zhong, Xueping. *Masculinity Besieged? Issues of Modernity and Male Subjectivity in Chinese Literature of the Late Twentieth Century.* Durham, N.C.: Duke University Press, 2000.

Zhongguo Zhongyi Yanjiuyuan Zhenjiu Yanjiu Suo Qigong Yanjiushi (Qigong research team, the Institute of Acupuncture, and Moxibustion, Academy of Traditional Chinese Medicine), ed. *Quanguo Ribaokan Qigong Wenxian Tilu: 1949–1986* (The index of qigong literature: 1949–1986). Beijing: Zhongguo Guji Chubanshe (Chinese ancient books press), 1988.

Zhu, Hong. "Women, Illness, and Hospitalization: Images in Contemporary Chinese Fiction." In *Engendering China: Women, Culture, and the State*, ed. Christina Gilmartin, Gail Hershatter, Lisa Rofel, and Tyrene White, 318–38. Cambridge: Harvard University Press, 1994.

Zhu, Xiaoyang. "Body and Soul in Ferment—China's Kungfu Craze." *Nexus China in Focus*, spring 1990, 4-12.

Zhuge, Xihan. *Di Er Jieguo Ji Qigong Hui Yixue Shu Lunwen Ji* (The collection of papers presented in the second international qigong studies conference). Xian, Shannxi Province: Tiance Chubanshe, 1989.

——. *Chaoren Zhang Baosheng* (Superman Zhang Baosheng). Guangzhou, Guangdong Province: Guangdong Renmin Chubanshe (Guangdong people's press), 1991.

Zito, Angela and Tani E. Barlow, eds. *Body, Subject, and Power in China*. Chicago: University of Chicago Press, 1994.

Zola, I. R. "Medicine as an Institution of Social Control." *Sociological Review* 20, no. 4 (1972): 487–504.

INDEX